Mometrix
TEST PREPARATION

I0889384

COCN®

Exam Secrets Study Guide

DEAR FUTURE EXAM SUCCESS STORY

First of all, **THANK YOU** for purchasing Mometrix study materials!

Second, congratulations! You are one of the few determined test-takers who are committed to doing whatever it takes to excel on your exam. **You have come to the right place.** We developed these study materials with one goal in mind: to deliver you the information you need in a format that's concise and easy to use.

In addition to optimizing your guide for the content of the test, we've outlined our recommended steps for breaking down the preparation process into small, attainable goals so you can make sure you stay on track.

We've also analyzed the entire test-taking process, identifying the most common pitfalls and showing how you can overcome them and be ready for any curveball the test throws you.

Standardized testing is one of the biggest obstacles on your road to success, which only increases the importance of doing well in the high-pressure, high-stakes environment of test day. Your results on this test could have a significant impact on your future, and this guide provides the information and practical advice to help you achieve your full potential on test day.

Your success is our success

We would love to hear from you! If you would like to share the story of your exam success or if you have any questions or comments in regard to our products, please contact us at **800-673-8175** or **support@mometrix.com**.

Thanks again for your business and we wish you continued success!

Sincerely,
The Mometrix Test Preparation Team

Need more help? Check out our flashcards at:
http://MometrixFlashcards.com/WOCNCB

Table of Contents

Introduction

Thank you for purchasing this resource! You have made the choice to prepare yourself for a test that could have a huge impact on your future, and this guide is designed to help you be fully ready for test day. Obviously, it's important to have a solid understanding of the test material, but you also need to be prepared for the unique environment and stressors of the test, so that you can perform to the best of your abilities.

For this purpose, the first section that appears in this guide is the **Secret Keys**. We've devoted countless hours to meticulously researching what works and what doesn't, and we've boiled down our findings to the five most impactful steps you can take to improve your performance on the test. We start at the beginning with study planning and move through the preparation process, all the way to the testing strategies that will help you get the most out of what you know when you're finally sitting in front of the test.

We recommend that you start preparing for your test as far in advance as possible. However, if you've bought this guide as a last-minute study resource and only have a few days before your test, we recommend that you skip over the first two Secret Keys since they address a long-term study plan.

If you struggle with **test anxiety**, we strongly encourage you to check out our recommendations for how you can overcome it. Test anxiety is a formidable foe, but it can be beaten, and we want to make sure you have the tools you need to defeat it.

Secret Key #1 – Plan Big, Study Small

There's a lot riding on your performance. If you want to ace this test, you're going to need to keep your skills sharp and the material fresh in your mind. You need a plan that lets you review everything you need to know while still fitting in your schedule. We'll break this strategy down into three categories.

Information Organization

Start with the information you already have: the official test outline. From this, you can make a complete list of all the concepts you need to cover before the test. Organize these concepts into groups that can be studied together, and create a list of any related vocabulary you need to learn so you can brush up on any difficult terms. You'll want to keep this vocabulary list handy once you actually start studying since you may need to add to it along the way.

Time Management

Once you have your set of study concepts, decide how to spread them out over the time you have left before the test. Break your study plan into small, clear goals so you have a manageable task for each day and know exactly what you're doing. Then just focus on one small step at a time. When you manage your time this way, you don't need to spend hours at a time studying. Studying a small block of content for a short period each day helps you retain information better and avoid stressing over how much you have left to do. You can relax knowing that you have a plan to cover everything in time. In order for this strategy to be effective though, you have to start studying early and stick to your schedule. Avoid the exhaustion and futility that comes from last-minute cramming!

Study Environment

The environment you study in has a big impact on your learning. Studying in a coffee shop, while probably more enjoyable, is not likely to be as fruitful as studying in a quiet room. It's important to keep distractions to a minimum. You're only planning to study for a short block of time, so make the most of it. Don't pause to check your phone or get up to find a snack. It's also important to **avoid multitasking**. Research has consistently shown that multitasking will make your studying dramatically less effective. Your study area should also be comfortable and well-lit so you don't have the distraction of straining your eyes or sitting on an uncomfortable chair.

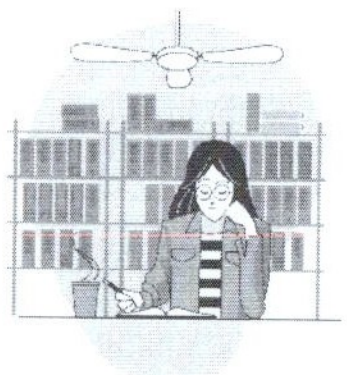

The time of day you study is also important. You want to be rested and alert. Don't wait until just before bedtime. Study when you'll be most likely to comprehend and remember. Even better, if you know what time of day your test will be, set that time aside for study. That way your brain will be used to working on that subject at that specific time and you'll have a better chance of recalling information.

Finally, it can be helpful to team up with others who are studying for the same test. Your actual studying should be done in as isolated an environment as possible, but the work of organizing the information and setting up the study plan can be divided up. In between study sessions, you can discuss with your teammates the concepts that you're all studying and quiz each other on the details. Just be sure that your teammates are as serious about the test as you are. If you find that your study time is being replaced with social time, you might need to find a new team.

Secret Key #2 – Make Your Studying Count

You're devoting a lot of time and effort to preparing for this test, so you want to be absolutely certain it will pay off. This means doing more than just reading the content and hoping you can remember it on test day. It's important to make every minute of study count. There are two main areas you can focus on to make your studying count.

Retention

It doesn't matter how much time you study if you can't remember the material. You need to make sure you are retaining the concepts. To check your retention of the information you're learning, try recalling it at later times with minimal prompting. Try carrying around flashcards and glance at one or two from time to time or ask a friend who's also studying for the test to quiz you.

To enhance your retention, look for ways to put the information into practice so that you can apply it rather than simply recalling it. If you're using the information in practical ways, it will be much easier to remember. Similarly, it helps to solidify a concept in your mind if you're not only reading it to yourself but also explaining it to someone else. Ask a friend to let you teach them about a concept you're a little shaky on (or speak aloud to an imaginary audience if necessary). As you try to summarize, define, give examples, and answer your friend's questions, you'll understand the concepts better and they will stay with you longer. Finally, step back for a big picture view and ask yourself how each piece of information fits with the whole subject. When you link the different concepts together and see them working together as a whole, it's easier to remember the individual components.

Finally, practice showing your work on any multi-step problems, even if you're just studying. Writing out each step you take to solve a problem will help solidify the process in your mind, and you'll be more likely to remember it during the test.

Modality

Modality simply refers to the means or method by which you study. Choosing a study modality that fits your own individual learning style is crucial. No two people learn best in exactly the same way, so it's important to know your strengths and use them to your advantage.

For example, if you learn best by visualization, focus on visualizing a concept in your mind and draw an image or a diagram. Try color-coding your notes, illustrating them, or creating symbols that will trigger your mind to recall a learned concept. If you learn best by hearing or discussing information, find a study partner who learns the same way or read aloud to yourself. Think about how to put the information in your own words. Imagine that you are giving a lecture on the topic and record yourself so you can listen to it later.

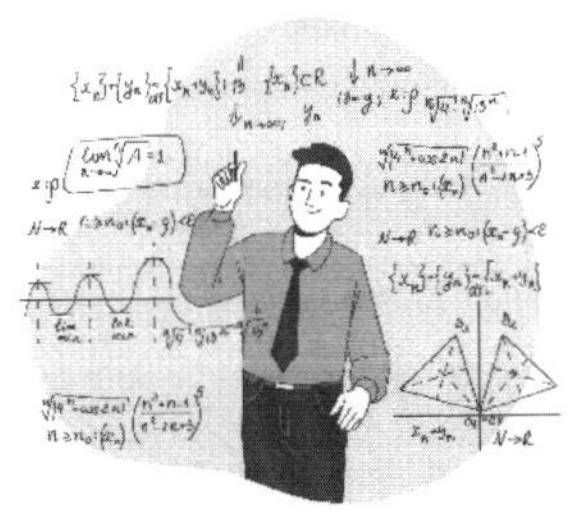

For any learning style, flashcards can be helpful. Organize the information so you can take advantage of spare moments to review. Underline key words or phrases. Use different colors for different categories. Mnemonic devices (such as creating a short list in which every item starts with the same letter) can also help with retention. Find what works best for you and use it to store the information in your mind most effectively and easily.

Secret Key #3 – Practice the Right Way

Your success on test day depends not only on how many hours you put into preparing, but also on whether you prepared the right way. It's good to check along the way to see if your studying is paying off. One of the most effective ways to do this is by taking practice tests to evaluate your progress. Practice tests are useful because they show exactly where you need to improve. Every time you take a practice test, pay special attention to these three groups of questions:

- The questions you got wrong
- The questions you had to guess on, even if you guessed right
- The questions you found difficult or slow to work through

This will show you exactly what your weak areas are, and where you need to devote more study time. Ask yourself why each of these questions gave you trouble. Was it because you didn't understand the material? Was it because you didn't remember the vocabulary? Do you need more repetitions on this type of question to build speed and confidence? Dig into those questions and figure out how you can strengthen your weak areas as you go back to review the material.

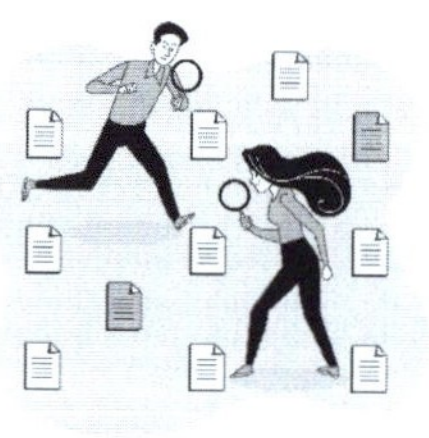

Additionally, many practice tests have a section explaining the answer choices. It can be tempting to read the explanation and think that you now have a good understanding of the concept. However, an explanation likely only covers part of the question's broader context. Even if the explanation makes perfect sense, **go back and investigate** every concept related to the question until you're positive you have a thorough understanding.

As you go along, keep in mind that the practice test is just that: practice. Memorizing these questions and answers will not be very helpful on the actual test because it is unlikely to have any of the same exact questions. If you only know the right answers to the sample questions, you won't be prepared for the real thing. **Study the concepts** until you understand them fully, and then you'll be able to answer any question that shows up on the test.

It's important to wait on the practice tests until you're ready. If you take a test on your first day of study, you may be overwhelmed by the amount of material covered and how much you need to learn. Work up to it gradually.

On test day, you'll need to be prepared for answering questions, managing your time, and using the test-taking strategies you've learned. It's a lot to balance, like a mental marathon that will have a big impact on your future. Like training for a marathon, you'll need to start slowly and work your way up. When test day arrives, you'll be ready.

Start with the strategies you've read in the first two Secret Keys—plan your course and study in the way that works best for you. If you have time, consider using multiple study resources to get different approaches to the same concepts. It can be helpful to see difficult concepts from more than one angle. Then find a good source for practice tests. Many times, the test website will suggest potential study resources or provide sample tests.

Practice Test Strategy

If you're able to find at least three practice tests, we recommend this strategy:

Untimed and Open-Book Practice

Take the first test with no time constraints and with your notes and study guide handy. Take your time and focus on applying the strategies you've learned.

Timed and Open-Book Practice

Take the second practice test open-book as well, but set a timer and practice pacing yourself to finish in time.

Timed and Closed-Book Practice

Take any other practice tests as if it were test day. Set a timer and put away your study materials. Sit at a table or desk in a quiet room, imagine yourself at the testing center, and answer questions as quickly and accurately as possible.

Keep repeating timed and closed-book tests on a regular basis until you run out of practice tests or it's time for the actual test. Your mind will be ready for the schedule and stress of test day, and you'll be able to focus on recalling the material you've learned.

Secret Key #4 – Pace Yourself

Once you're fully prepared for the material on the test, your biggest challenge on test day will be managing your time. Just knowing that the clock is ticking can make you panic even if you have plenty of time left. Work on pacing yourself so you can build confidence against the time constraints of the exam. Pacing is a difficult skill to master, especially in a high-pressure environment, so **practice is vital**.

Set time expectations for your pace based on how much time is available. For example, if a section has 60 questions and the time limit is 30 minutes, you know you have to average 30 seconds or less per question in order to answer them all. Although 30 seconds is the hard limit, set 25 seconds per question as your goal, so you reserve extra time to spend on harder questions. When you budget extra time for the harder questions, you no longer have any reason to stress when those questions take longer to answer.

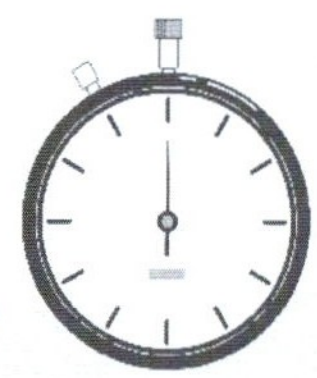

Don't let this time expectation distract you from working through the test at a calm, steady pace, but keep it in mind so you don't spend too much time on any one question. Recognize that taking extra time on one question you don't understand may keep you from answering two that you do understand later in the test. If your time limit for a question is up and you're still not sure of the answer, mark it and move on, and come back to it later if the time and the test format allow. If the testing format doesn't allow you to return to earlier questions, just make an educated guess; then put it out of your mind and move on.

On the easier questions, be careful not to rush. It may seem wise to hurry through them so you have more time for the challenging ones, but it's not worth missing one if you know the concept and just didn't take the time to read the question fully. Work efficiently but make sure you understand the question and have looked at all of the answer choices, since more than one may seem right at first.

Even if you're paying attention to the time, you may find yourself a little behind at some point. You should speed up to get back on track, but do so wisely. Don't panic; just take a few seconds less on each question until you're caught up. Don't guess without thinking, but do look through the answer choices and eliminate any you know are wrong. If you can get down to two choices, it is often worthwhile to guess from those. Once you've chosen an answer, move on and don't dwell on any that you skipped or had to hurry through. If a question was taking too long, chances are it was one of the harder ones, so you weren't as likely to get it right anyway.

On the other hand, if you find yourself getting ahead of schedule, it may be beneficial to slow down a little. The more quickly you work, the more likely you are to make a careless mistake that will affect your score. You've budgeted time for each question, so don't be afraid to spend that time. Practice an efficient but careful pace to get the most out of the time you have.

Secret Key #5 – Have a Plan for Guessing

When you're taking the test, you may find yourself stuck on a question. Some of the answer choices seem better than others, but you don't see the one answer choice that is obviously correct. What do you do?

The scenario described above is very common, yet most test takers have not effectively prepared for it. Developing and practicing a plan for guessing may be one of the single most effective uses of your time as you get ready for the exam.

In developing your plan for guessing, there are three questions to address:

- When should you start the guessing process?
- How should you narrow down the choices?
- Which answer should you choose?

When to Start the Guessing Process

Unless your plan for guessing is to select C every time (which, despite its merits, is not what we recommend), you need to leave yourself enough time to apply your answer elimination strategies. Since you have a limited amount of time for each question, that means that if you're going to give yourself the best shot at guessing correctly, you have to decide quickly whether or not you will guess.

Of course, the best-case scenario is that you don't have to guess at all, so first, see if you can answer the question based on your knowledge of the subject and basic reasoning skills. Focus on the key words in the question and try to jog your memory of related topics. Give yourself a chance to bring the knowledge to mind, but once you realize that you don't have (or you can't access) the knowledge you need to answer the question, it's time to start the guessing process.

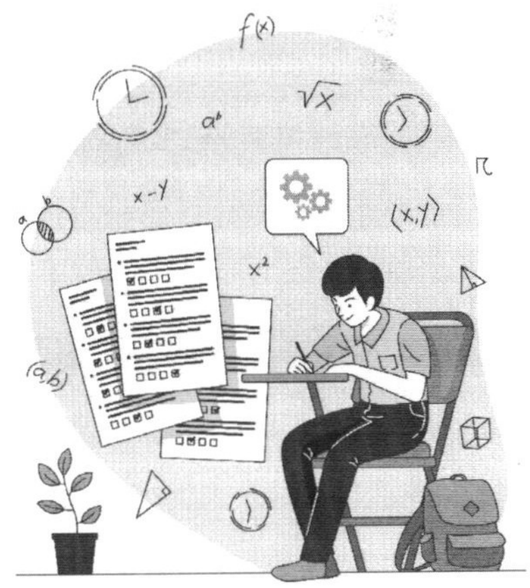

It's almost always better to start the guessing process too early than too late. It only takes a few seconds to remember something and answer the question from knowledge. Carefully eliminating wrong answer choices takes longer. Plus, going through the process of eliminating answer choices can actually help jog your memory.

Summary: Start the guessing process as soon as you decide that you can't answer the question based on your knowledge.

How to Narrow Down the Choices

The next chapter in this book (**Test-Taking Strategies**) includes a wide range of strategies for how to approach questions and how to look for answer choices to eliminate. You will definitely want to read those carefully, practice them, and figure out which ones work best for you. Here though, we're going to address a mindset rather than a particular strategy.

Your odds of guessing an answer correctly depend on how many options you are choosing from.

Number of options left	5	4	3	2	1
Odds of guessing correctly	20%	25%	33%	50%	100%

You can see from this chart just how valuable it is to be able to eliminate incorrect answers and make an educated guess, but there are two things that many test takers do that cause them to miss out on the benefits of guessing:

- Accidentally eliminating the correct answer
- Selecting an answer based on an impression

We'll look at the first one here, and the second one in the next section.

To avoid accidentally eliminating the correct answer, we recommend a thought exercise called **the $5 challenge**. In this challenge, you only eliminate an answer choice from contention if you are willing to bet $5 on it being wrong. Why $5? Five dollars is a small but not insignificant amount of money. It's an amount you could afford to lose but wouldn't want to throw away. And while losing $5 once might not hurt too much, doing it twenty times will set you back $100. In the same way, each small decision you make—eliminating a choice here, guessing on a question there—won't by itself impact your score very much, but when you put them all together, they can make a big difference. By holding each answer choice elimination decision to a higher standard, you can reduce the risk of accidentally eliminating the correct answer.

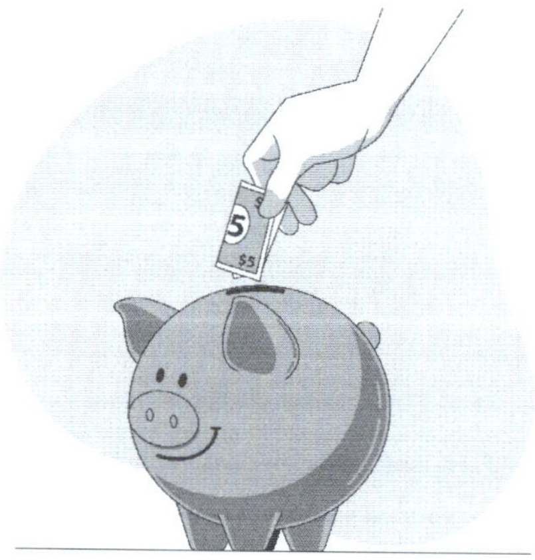

The $5 challenge can also be applied in a positive sense: If you are willing to bet $5 that an answer choice *is* correct, go ahead and mark it as correct.

Summary: Only eliminate an answer choice if you are willing to bet $5 that it is wrong.

Which Answer to Choose

You're taking the test. You've run into a hard question and decided you'll have to guess. You've eliminated all the answer choices you're willing to bet $5 on. Now you have to pick an answer. Why do we even need to talk about this? Why can't you just pick whichever one you feel like when the time comes?

The answer to these questions is that if you don't come into the test with a plan, you'll rely on your impression to select an answer choice, and if you do that, you risk falling into a trap. The test writers know that everyone who takes their test will be guessing on some of the questions, so they intentionally write wrong answer choices to seem plausible. You still have to pick an answer though, and if the wrong answer choices are designed to look right, how can you ever be sure that you're not falling for their trap? The best solution we've found to this dilemma is to take the decision out of your hands entirely. Here is the process we recommend:

Once you've eliminated any choices that you are confident (willing to bet $5) are wrong, select the first remaining choice as your answer.

Whether you choose to select the first remaining choice, the second, or the last, the important thing is that you use some preselected standard. Using this approach guarantees that you will not be enticed into selecting an answer choice that looks right, because you are not basing your decision on how the answer choices look.

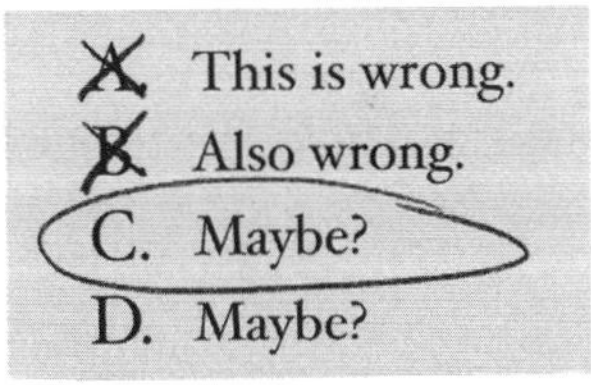

This is not meant to make you question your knowledge. Instead, it is to help you recognize the difference between your knowledge and your impressions. There's a huge difference between thinking an answer is right because of what you know, and thinking an answer is right because it looks or sounds like it should be right.

Summary: To ensure that your selection is appropriately random, make a predetermined selection from among all answer choices you have not eliminated.

Test-Taking Strategies

This section contains a list of test-taking strategies that you may find helpful as you work through the test. By taking what you know and applying logical thought, you can maximize your chances of answering any question correctly!

It is very important to realize that every question is different and every person is different: no single strategy will work on every question, and no single strategy will work for every person. That's why we've included all of them here, so you can try them out and determine which ones work best for different types of questions and which ones work best for you.

Question Strategies

✓ Read Carefully

Read the question and the answer choices carefully. Don't miss the question because you misread the terms. You have plenty of time to read each question thoroughly and make sure you understand what is being asked. Yet a happy medium must be attained, so don't waste too much time. You must read carefully and efficiently.

✓ Contextual Clues

Look for contextual clues. If the question includes a word you are not familiar with, look at the immediate context for some indication of what the word might mean. Contextual clues can often give you all the information you need to decipher the meaning of an unfamiliar word. Even if you can't determine the meaning, you may be able to narrow down the possibilities enough to make a solid guess at the answer to the question.

✓ Prefixes

If you're having trouble with a word in the question or answer choices, try dissecting it. Take advantage of every clue that the word might include. Prefixes can be a huge help. Usually, they allow you to determine a basic meaning. *Pre-* means before, *post-* means after, *pro-* is positive, *de-* is negative. From prefixes, you can get an idea of the general meaning of the word and try to put it into context.

✓ Hedge Words

Watch out for critical hedge words, such as *likely, may, can, often, almost, mostly, usually, generally, rarely,* and *sometimes.* Question writers insert these hedge phrases to cover every possibility. Often an answer choice will be wrong simply because it leaves no room for exception. Be on guard for answer choices that have definitive words such as *exactly* and *always.*

✓ Switchback Words

Stay alert for *switchbacks.* These are the words and phrases frequently used to alert you to shifts in thought. The most common switchback words are *but, although,* and *however.* Others include *nevertheless, on the other hand, even though, while, in spite of, despite,* and *regardless of.* Switchback words are important to catch because they can change the direction of the question or an answer choice.

✓ FACE VALUE

When in doubt, use common sense. Accept the situation in the problem at face value. Don't read too much into it. These problems will not require you to make wild assumptions. If you have to go beyond creativity and warp time or space in order to have an answer choice fit the question, then you should move on and consider the other answer choices. These are normal problems rooted in reality. The applicable relationship or explanation may not be readily apparent, but it is there for you to figure out. Use your common sense to interpret anything that isn't clear.

Answer Choice Strategies

✓ ANSWER SELECTION

The most thorough way to pick an answer choice is to identify and eliminate wrong answers until only one is left, then confirm it is the correct answer. Sometimes an answer choice may immediately seem right, but be careful. The test writers will usually put more than one reasonable answer choice on each question, so take a second to read all of them and make sure that the other choices are not equally obvious. As long as you have time left, it is better to read every answer choice than to pick the first one that looks right without checking the others.

✓ ANSWER CHOICE FAMILIES

An answer choice family consists of two (in rare cases, three) answer choices that are very similar in construction and cannot all be true at the same time. If you see two answer choices that are direct opposites or parallels, one of them is usually the correct answer. For instance, if one answer choice says that quantity *x* increases and another either says that quantity *x* decreases (opposite) or says that quantity *y* increases (parallel), then those answer choices would fall into the same family. An answer choice that doesn't match the construction of the answer choice family is more likely to be incorrect. Most questions will not have answer choice families, but when they do appear, you should be prepared to recognize them.

✓ ELIMINATE ANSWERS

Eliminate answer choices as soon as you realize they are wrong, but make sure you consider all possibilities. If you are eliminating answer choices and realize that the last one you are left with is also wrong, don't panic. Start over and consider each choice again. There may be something you missed the first time that you will realize on the second pass.

✓ AVOID FACT TRAPS

Don't be distracted by an answer choice that is factually true but doesn't answer the question. You are looking for the choice that answers the question. Stay focused on what the question is asking for so you don't accidentally pick an answer that is true but incorrect. Always go back to the question and make sure the answer choice you've selected actually answers the question and is not merely a true statement.

✓ EXTREME STATEMENTS

In general, you should avoid answers that put forth extreme actions as standard practice or proclaim controversial ideas as established fact. An answer choice that states the "process should be used in certain situations, if…" is much more likely to be correct than one that states the "process should be discontinued completely." The first is a calm rational statement and doesn't even make a definitive, uncompromising stance, using a hedge word *if* to provide wiggle room, whereas the second choice is far more extreme.

☑ BENCHMARK

As you read through the answer choices and you come across one that seems to answer the question well, mentally select that answer choice. This is not your final answer, but it's the one that will help you evaluate the other answer choices. The one that you selected is your benchmark or standard for judging each of the other answer choices. Every other answer choice must be compared to your benchmark. That choice is correct until proven otherwise by another answer choice beating it. If you find a better answer, then that one becomes your new benchmark. Once you've decided that no other choice answers the question as well as your benchmark, you have your final answer.

☑ PREDICT THE ANSWER

Before you even start looking at the answer choices, it is often best to try to predict the answer. When you come up with the answer on your own, it is easier to avoid distractions and traps because you will know exactly what to look for. The right answer choice is unlikely to be word-for-word what you came up with, but it should be a close match. Even if you are confident that you have the right answer, you should still take the time to read each option before moving on.

General Strategies

☑ TOUGH QUESTIONS

If you are stumped on a problem or it appears too hard or too difficult, don't waste time. Move on! Remember though, if you can quickly check for obviously incorrect answer choices, your chances of guessing correctly are greatly improved. Before you completely give up, at least try to knock out a couple of possible answers. Eliminate what you can and then guess at the remaining answer choices before moving on.

☑ CHECK YOUR WORK

Since you will probably not know every term listed and the answer to every question, it is important that you get credit for the ones that you do know. Don't miss any questions through careless mistakes. If at all possible, try to take a second to look back over your answer selection and make sure you've selected the correct answer choice and haven't made a costly careless mistake (such as marking an answer choice that you didn't mean to mark). This quick double check should more than pay for itself in caught mistakes for the time it costs.

☑ PACE YOURSELF

It's easy to be overwhelmed when you're looking at a page full of questions; your mind is confused and full of random thoughts, and the clock is ticking down faster than you would like. Calm down and maintain the pace that you have set for yourself. Especially as you get down to the last few minutes of the test, don't let the small numbers on the clock make you panic. As long as you are on track by monitoring your pace, you are guaranteed to have time for each question.

☑ DON'T RUSH

It is very easy to make errors when you are in a hurry. Maintaining a fast pace in answering questions is pointless if it makes you miss questions that you would have gotten right otherwise. Test writers like to include distracting information and wrong answers that seem right. Taking a little extra time to avoid careless mistakes can make all the difference in your test score. Find a pace that allows you to be confident in the answers that you select.

✓ KEEP MOVING

Panicking will not help you pass the test, so do your best to stay calm and keep moving. Taking deep breaths and going through the answer elimination steps you practiced can help to break through a stress barrier and keep your pace.

Final Notes

The combination of a solid foundation of content knowledge and the confidence that comes from practicing your plan for applying that knowledge is the key to maximizing your performance on test day. As your foundation of content knowledge is built up and strengthened, you'll find that the strategies included in this chapter become more and more effective in helping you quickly sift through the distractions and traps of the test to isolate the correct answer.

Now that you're preparing to move forward into the test content chapters of this book, be sure to keep your goal in mind. As you read, think about how you will be able to apply this information on the test. If you've already seen sample questions for the test and you have an idea of the question format and style, try to come up with questions of your own that you can answer based on what you're reading. This will give you valuable practice applying your knowledge in the same ways you can expect to on test day.

Good luck and good studying!

Assessment and Care Planning

Etiology, Risk Factors, and Screening

ANATOMY OF THE GASTROINTESTINAL SYSTEM

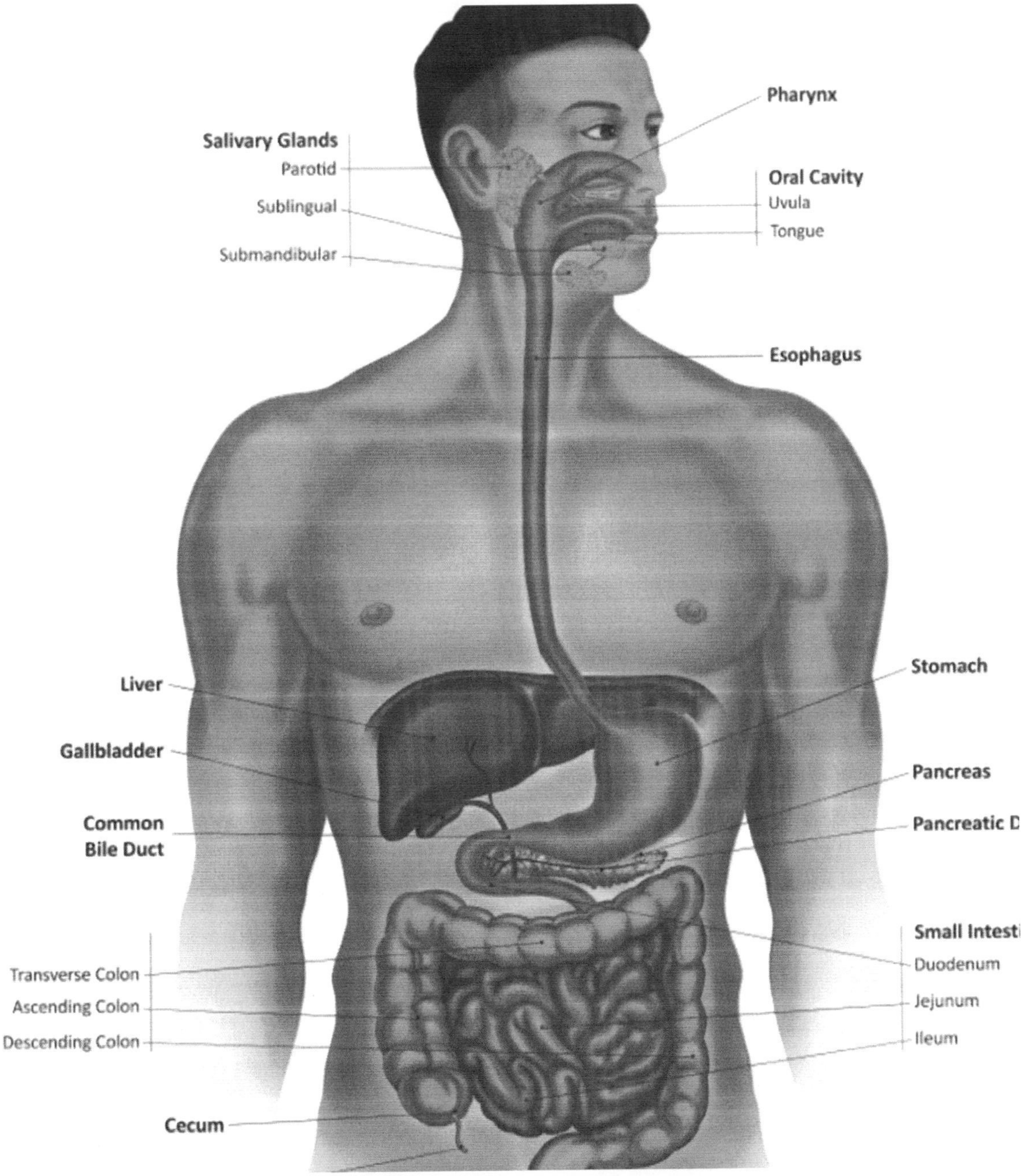

Anatomy of the Genitourinary System

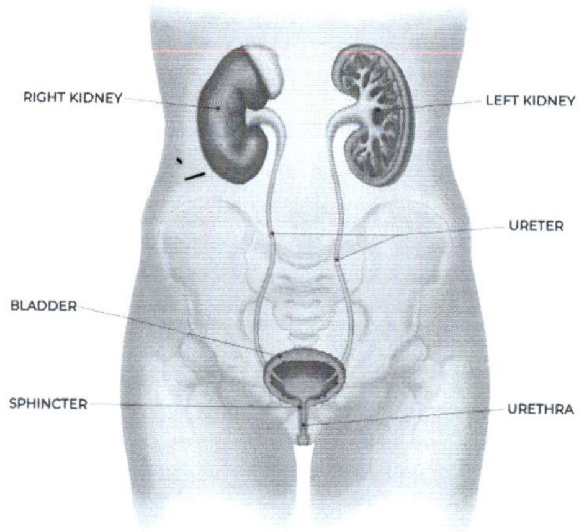

Urinary Incontinence

The different types of urinary incontinence are as follows:

- **Urge**: An urgency to urinate as soon as the bladder feels full, so person may urinate on the way to the toilet or in bed during the night. Diuretics may exacerbate urge incontinence.
- **Stress**: A sudden increase in bladder pressure from things such as coughing, laughing, or bending causes small amount of urinary leakage. It is common in people who are obese.
- **Overflow**: An overfull bladder causes dribbling of urine, usually in small amounts but the leakage can be almost constant.
- **Functional**: Incontinence caused by physical or mental impairment, such as dementia. May also be related to environmental barriers to urination, such as no accessible bathroom.
- **Reflex**: Loss of urine takes place without awareness of person because of fistula or bladder leak.
- **Mixed**: There may be more than one type of incontinence.
- **Induced**: Some surgical procedures (hysterectomy, prostatectomy, rectal surgery) can damage nerves or muscles that control urination.

Right-Sided (Ascending) Colon Cancer

Stool enters the cecum and ascending colon in liquid form, so cancers arising in these areas may grow to a large size before they cause obstruction and obvious symptoms. Lesions frequently grow into the lumen of the intestine and ulcerate, causing chronic bleeding that may not change the character or the appearance of stool. Liquid stool can pass through even a very narrow opening. 20% of colorectal tumors arise in the ascending colon.

Symptoms include:

- Fatigue: Generalized weakness.
- Pallor: Dull abdominal pain.
- Anorexia: Unexplained weight loss.
- Occult blood or melena (tarry stools).
- Hypochromic microcytic anemia.
- Chronic iron deficiency anemia.

- Palpitations or congestive heart failure related to anemia.
- Palpable abdominal mass may be evident with large tumors.
- Chronic diarrhea may rarely develop with some large right-sided lesions.
- Obstruction may occur in late stages.

TNM Staging for Adenocarcinoma of the Colon

Tumor, node, metastasis (TNM) staging is one method of staging cancer by examining the extent of the tumor, extent of lymph node involvement, and whether the cancer has metastasized. The scoring of each of those components combine to equate to the cancer's staging.

- **Stage 0**: Cancer cells are found in the lining of the intestine but have not spread to the outer layers or spread to the lymph nodes (carcinoma in situ).
- **Stage I**: Cancer has spread from the lining of the intestine into the submucosa layer and may extend into the muscle layer, but has not yet spread to the lymph nodes.
- **Stage II**: Cancer has spread to the muscle layer, the serosa, and invaded adjacent tissue, but has not yet spread to the lymph nodes.
- **Stage III**: Cancer has invaded all layers of the intestine, spread into adjacent tissue, and invaded some regional lymph nodes. The cancer has not spread to distant lymph nodes or organs.
- **Stage IV**: Cancer has spread, or metastasized, to other parts of the body, such as the liver, lungs, brain, or bones, with or without spread to the lymph nodes.

Diagnostic Testing for Bladder Cancer, Interstitial Cystitis, Refractory Radiation Cystitis, Neurogenic Bladder, and Prostate Cancer

Diagnostics for bladder cancer, interstitial cystitis, and refractory radiation cystitis include:

- **Urinalysis** identifies hematuria or other abnormalities of the urinary tract.
- **Urine culture** rules out or identifies infectious agents.
- Electrolytes, BUN, creatinine evaluates renal function.
- **CT scan/ultrasound** identifies cause of hematuria or other symptoms and identifies lesions.
- **Intravenous Pyelogram** identifies abnormalities within the entire urinary tract and rules out other causes of hematuria.
- **Cystoscopy** confirms a diagnosis, rules out other diseases, and views the type and extent of lesions.
- **Biopsy** determines the tumor grade and depth of lesion.

Diagnostics for neurogenic bladder include:

- **24-hour urine collection** determines volume and urine patterns.
- **Bladder stress test** determines reaction to full bladder while bending over, coughing, walking, or doing other activities.

Diagnostics for prostate cancer include:

- **Prostate-specific antigen test (PSA)** determines if cancer of the prostate has blocked the prostate ducts, causing an increase in blood levels of PSA.

American Cancer Society's Risk Factors for Bladder Cancer

The American Cancer Society's risk factors for bladder cancer are as follows:

- **Smoking**: greatest risk factor; smokers have twice bladder cancer as nonsmokers. Carcinogens in lungs enter blood stream, are filtered by kidneys, and concentrated in urine, damaging bladder lining.
- **Occupational hazards**: exposure to aniline dye and aromatic amines and other organic chemicals.
- **Race**: Caucasians twice as likely to develop bladder cancer.
- **Age**: over 70% are over 65 years old.
- **Gender**: rate for men is 4 times that of women.
- **Chronic bladder inflammation**: especially with indwelling catheters or bladders left intact after urinary diversion.
- Previous bladder cancer: possible recurrence.
- **Congenital defects**: retention of urachus (connection between umbilicus and bladder) after birth. Exstrophy, defect in the bladder wall.
- **Genetics**: family clusters occur.
- **Chemotherapy/radiation**: high doses of cyclophosphamide and ifosfamide and radiation to pelvis.
- **Arsenic in drinking water**: risk depends upon water system meeting standards for arsenic consumption.
- **Low fluid consumption**: keeps chemicals in urine in contact with bladder.
- **Parasites**: schistosomiasis, worms lay eggs in muscle wall of bladder, causing chronic irritation.

Bladder Cancer

Bladder cancer and most other urinary cancers begin in the inside lining of the urinary organs and then invade the deeper layers. The bladder wall and lining of urinary tract consist of several layers, from the inside wall to the outside lining:

- **Urothelium** (mucosa): Urothelial (transitional) cells line the inside layer of the urinary tract.
- **Lamina propria** (sub-mucosa): Thin layer of connective tissue.
- **Muscularis propria** (muscular): Thicker layer of muscle.
- **Serosa**: Fatty connective tissue covers superior surfaces.
- **Adventitia**: Covers areas with no serosa.

Symptoms include:

- **Gross hematuria**: Frank bright red blood may be evident. Sometimes urine brown or rust-colored. This is usually the first sign of bladder cancer. Blood in urine may appear, disappear, and reappear, usually without pain.
- **Microscopic hematuria**: Blood may be present but only visible under microscope examination.
- **Dysuria**: May have burning on urination or pain as well as feeling that bladder does not completely empty on urination, and frequency.

TYPES OF BLADDER CANCER AND CANCERS OF LINING OF OTHER URINARY ORGANS

Urothelial carcinoma: Cancer of urothelial (transitional) cells cause over 90% of these cancers, classified into subtypes:

- **Non-invasive**: Only in urothelium.
- **Invasive**: Spreads from urothelium to deeper layers.
- **Superficial**: Invasive and noninvasive cancers that have not spread or only invaded the lamina propria.
- **Flat**: Only grow in wall and may be noninvasive carcinoma affecting inner layer or invasive invading the deep layers, particularly the muscularis propria.
- **Papillary**: Tumors with finger-like projections usually growing into hollow center of bladder. Classified into subtypes:
  - Noninvasive: Only grow into center of bladder:
  - Papillomas: Benign.
  - Neoplasms: Low malignancy but may recur in more malignant form.
  - Carcinomas: Low grade rarely invade bladder wall but often recur; high grade may invade bladder wall and metastasize.
  - Invasive: Grow toward center and into wall.

Squamous cell carcinoma: Causes 4% of cancers, usually invasive.

Adenocarcinoma: Causes 1-2% of cancers; similar to intestinal cancers, invasive.

Small cell: Causes about 1% of cancers.

INTERSTITIAL CYSTITIS

Interstitial cystitis (painful bladder syndrome) causes chronic debilitating pain of bladder, urethra, and pelvic area as well as dysuria. May relate to congenital or traumatic injuries that cause inflammation and problems with urine storage and bladder emptying. The underlying cause is not known at this time. Does not respond to antibiotic therapy. Pain may persist after surgery. Affects women over men 9:1.

Symptoms include:

- Pain from mild to severe.
- Urgency.
- Frequency.
- The bladder wall may be irritated and scarred.
- Hunner's ulcers of bladder wall mucosa may occur.
- Glomerulations (pinpoint bleeding) on bladder wall.

Diagnosis is by:

- **Urinalysis**: To identify hematuria or other abnormalities of the urinary tract.
- **Urine culture**: To rule out or identify infectious agents.
- **Cystoscopy**: To confirm a diagnosis, rule out other diseases, and view the type and extent of lesions. Procedure done under anesthesia may include testing of maximum bladder capacity.
- **Biopsy**: To evaluate bladder wall.

Treatments for interstitial cystitis:

- Bladder distention sometimes relieves symptoms.
- Bladder instillation with dimethyl sulfoxide (DMSO) uses catheter to instill medication that is held for 15 minutes. Treatments every 1-2 weeks for 6-8 weeks and repeated as needed. May be self administered.
- Medications may give relief: ASA, ibuprofen, pentosan polysulfate sodium (Elmiron).
- Transcutaneous electrical nerve stimulation (TENS) to lower back or above pubic area may relieve pelvic pain.
- Diet may affect pain. Elimination and reintroduction of foods can help to identify those exacerbating pain.
- Bladder training includes maintaining diary and scheduled voiding, gradually lengthening time between urinations.
- **Surgery** with different options available:
  - **Fulguration**: Cystoscopic cauterizing of Hunner's ulcers to promote sloughing and healing.
  - **Resection**: Cystoscopic resection of ulcers.
  - **Bladder augmentation/reconstruction**: Ulcerated and inflamed tissue removed and piece of colon removed, shaped, and used to form part of bladder wall.
- Cystectomy with urinary diversion: If other treatments fail.

Refractory Radiation Cystitis

Refractory radiation cystitis: Damage from radiation of pelvic tumors resulting in intractable incontinence or urinary fistulas. Radiation may damage the bladder muscle or sphincter. This condition may relate to primary radiation for treatment of bladder cancer or incidental radiation from treatment of cancer in proximal areas. Treatment with both radiation and chemotherapy can increase the risk of developing this disorder. Radiation can cause damage to vessels, and deposits of collagen may result in scarring with further damage to blood vessel, which can result in tissue hypoxia and necrosis.

Symptoms may vary depending upon the degree of damage to the tissue. Early symptoms relate to submucosal inflammation, fibrosis, and ulcerations. Later symptoms related to occlusion of lumens, vascular ectasia (thinning), and vessel wall necrosis.

- **Acute/early**: Urgency, frequency, hematuria, dysuria.
- **Chronic/late**: Worsening of early symptoms and ischemia and fibrosis, leading to ulceration, fistulas, fecaluria, hydronephrosis, and incontinence.

Diagnostic Procedures and Treatments

Tests are done to rule out other disorders:

- **Urinalysis**: To identify hematuria or other abnormalities.
- **Complete blood count**: To evaluate anemia/infection.
- **Urine culture**: To rule out/identify infectious agents.
- **Electrolytes, BUN, creatinine**: To evaluate renal function.
- **CT scan/ultrasound**: To identify cause of hematuria or other symptoms and identify lesions.
- **Intravenous pyelogram**: To identify abnormalities within the entire urinary tract and rule out other causes of hematuria.
- **Cystoscopy**: To confirm diagnosis, rule out other diseases, and view type and extent of lesions.

Medical management includes:

- **Anticholinergic agents**: Relieve frequency/urgency.
- **Conjugated estrogens**: Promote healing.
- **Hyperbaric oxygen therapy**: Repair vascular changes; will not reverse changes caused by significant fibrosis or ischemia. May preserve bladder function. Thirty treatments are usual.

Surgical management includes:

- **Cystoscopy with fulguration**: Treat lesions.
- **Percutaneous nephrostomy tube insertion**: Drain urine.
- **Bladder augmentation**: Correct small bladder.
- **Bladder irrigations and instillations**: Treat irritation.
- **Cystectomy with urinary diversion**: For severe cases non-responsive to medical treatment.

American Cancer Society's Risk Factors for Prostate Cancer

Risk factors for prostate cancer:

- **Age**: Risk increases after age 50 with two-thirds after 65.
- **Race**: African Americans are twice as likely to die of prostate cancer as Caucasians. Asians have the lowest rates for reasons unclear.
- **Nationality**: Most common in North America and northwestern Europe.
- **Family history**: Family clusters occur. A father or brother with prostate cancer doubles risk. Several affected relatives, especially with onset at early age, increases risk. Several inherited genes may increase risk, but genetic testing for these genes is not yet available.
- **Diet**: Diets high in red meat or high-fat dairy products with fewer fruits and vegetables may cause slight increased risk. Researchers are unsure which dietary factor raises risk.
- **Exercise**: Over age 65 may contribute to lower rate.
- **Vasectomy**: Research is inconclusive with some studies suggesting that men who have vasectomies before age 35 may have increased risk.

Small Intestine Cancer

The small bowel is part of the digestive tract, extending from the stomach to the colon. It is divided into three parts—duodenum, jejunum, and ileum—and is approximately 16 feet in length.

Types

The 4 main types of primary small intestine cancer are named for the type of cells from which they develop:

- **Adenocarcinomas**: Arise in lining of intestine and are the most common type, usually occurring in the duodenum.
- **Carcinoids**: Arise in hormone-producing cells in the small bowel, occurring most often in the ileum, but sometimes in the appendix.
- **Lymphomas**: Arise in the lymph tissue and are usually non-Hodgkin lymphomas, occurring most commonly in the jejunum or ileum.
- **Sarcomas**: Arise in the supportive tissues, such as fat and muscle. Leiomyosarcoma usually form in the muscle wall of the ileum. Gastrointestinal stromal tumors may develop in any part of the small intestine.

Symptoms

The **symptoms of cancer of the small intestine** develop as the tumor grows, disturbing the natural functioning of the bowel. Cancer is often non-specific and vague and may resemble those of other disorders, but often worsens over time and lasts for many weeks. It is most common in people over age 50:

- Blood loss
  - Blood in stools or tarry stools from partially digested blood.
  - Anemia may develop from chronic bleeding.
- Discomfort
  - Abdominal discomfort, cramping.
  - Palpable mass may be evident.
- Inflammation
  - Chronic or recurrent diarrhea may occur.
  - Weight loss without dieting from malabsorption.
- Anorexia
- Obstruction: Complete/partial obstruction may result as cancer spreads; may be intermittent if no inflammatory disease.
  - Constipation. Nausea and vomiting. Abdominal distension.
  - Severe pain.
- Perforation (from obstruction)
  - Severe, acute pain. Hypotensive shock.
  - Abdominal distension. Peritonitis may occur.

Colorectal Cancer

Risk Factors

Risk factors for colorectal cancer include the following:

- **Adenomatous polyps**, especially large or multiple, can become cancerous.
- **Age**: Over 90% of people with colorectal cancer are over 50.
- **Alcohol intake**, especially heavy use, is linked to colorectal cancer, possibly due to alcohol's effect on folic acid.
- **Diet high in animal fats**, especially red meat, and low in fiber is a risk factor.
- **Family history** of colorectal cancer in first-degree relatives (parents, siblings, and children) is a risk factor for about 30% of those with colorectal cancer.
- **Genetic disorders** are related to cancer:
- **Familial adenomatous polyposis** (FAP) causes about 1% of colorectal cancers. Are related to this syndrome.
- **Hereditary non-polyposis colorectal cancer** (HNPCC) causes about 3-5% of colorectal cancers.
- **Inflammatory bowel disease** (ulcerative colitis and Crohn's disease) can lead to cancer.
- **Personal history** of colorectal cancer predisposes to recurrence.
- **Smoking** may account for 12% of colorectal cancers. Cancer-causing substances in cigarettes are swallowed and enter the digestive system.

Screening

Screening recommendations for colorectal cancer (according to the CDC):

- Screening should begin at age 45 for individuals without risk factors.
- Screening should begin earlier, generally at age 40, if risk factors are present, such as:
    - Family history of colorectal cancer in first or second-degree relatives.
    - Family history of genetic syndrome (FAP, HNLPCC).
    - Adenomatous polyps in first-degree relatives before age 60.
    - History of polyps or colorectal cancer.
    - History of inflammatory bowel disease.

Types of screening tests include:

- **Fecal occult blood**—yearly: Checks for blood in stool.
- **Flexible sigmoidoscopy**—every 5 years, or every 10 years with a fecal immunochemical test (FIT) annually: Scope to check for polyps or signs of cancer in rectum and lower third of colon. (Often done with fecal occult blood test.)
- **Colonoscopy**—every 10 years or as follow-up for abnormalities in other screening: Longer flexible scope, usually with anesthesia, to check rectum and entire colon. It allows for removal of polyps, small cancerous lesions, and biopsies and provides surveillance of inflammatory bowel disease.
- **CT Colonography**—every 5 years: Digital scan using x-ray technology that captures images of the entire colon and displays them on the computer screen for analysis.

Diagnostic Testing

Diagnostic testing for colorectal cancer includes the following:

- **Full colonoscopy** is more accurate than flexible sigmoidoscopy and better able to confirm the location of tumor and facilitate tissue biopsy and removal of polyps.
- **Double contrast barium enema** is useful with colonoscopy for right-sided lesions.
- **Complete blood testing** may indicate anemia from local blood loss. Liver chemistries may show hepatic metastasis, especially elevation of alkaline phosphatase, and tumor markers may indicate advanced disease. Carcinoembryonic antigen (CEA) may be elevated with colorectal cancer.
- **Chest x-ray** is used to rule out lung metastasis.
- **CT scan of chest** is needed if x-ray positive for added information about extent of lesions. CT of pelvic and abdominal area remains controversial for colon cancer because it does not always show liver metastasis and doesn't stage well.
- **CT scan/MRI of pelvic and abdominal area** is used for rectal cancer to verify absence of obvious metastasis.
- **Endoluminal ultrasound (ELUS)** is used to stage rectal tumors and to show extent of tumor invasion.

Types

Types of colorectal cancer include:

- **Adenocarcinomas** develop from epithelial tissue in adenomatous polyps and account for 90-95% of all colorectal cancers. There are two sub-types:
- **Signet ring** is a very aggressive form that is harder to treat but accounts for only 0.1% of adenocarcinomas.
- **Mucinous** is also an aggressive form that is composed of about 60% mucous, allowing the cells to spread faster and making it hard to treat. This form accounts for 10-15% of adenocarcinomas.
- **Sarcomas (Leiomyosarcoma)** develop from smooth muscle and account for less than 2% of colorectal cancers, but over 50% metastasize.
- **Carcinoids** are slow-growing tumors that rarely spread, most commonly found in the rectum and accounting for less than 1% of colorectal cancers.
- **Lymphomas** are rare and primary tumors occurring primarily in rectum while secondary metastatic tumors occur primarily in the colon.
- **Melanomas** are rare tumors usually metastasize from other parts of body; accounts for less than 2% of colorectal cancers.

Dukes' Modified Staging Classification

The **Dukes' staging system's original three classes have been modified to 6.** While this staging is still used, the TNM (tumor, node, and metastasis) staging is more common.

- **Class A**: Tumor invades only the mucosa of intestinal wall.
- **Class B1**: Tumor invades the muscle layer (muscularis propria) of intestinal wall, but doesn't go all the way through.
- **Class B2**: Tumor invades and goes all the way through the muscle layer (muscularis propria) of intestinal wall.
- **Class C1**: As in B1, tumor invades the muscle layer of the intestinal wall but doesn't go all the way through; however, there is evidence of cancerous cells in the lymph nodes.

- **Class C2**: As in B2, tumor invades and goes all the way through the muscle layer; additionally, there is evidence of cancerous cells in the lymph nodes.
- **Class D**: Tumor has metastasized beyond the lymph nodes to organs, such as liver, bones, or lungs.

Transverse, Descending, Sigmoid, and Rectal Cancers

Because some of the fluid in intestines is absorbed in the ascending colon, stool in the transverse and descending colon is more formed. Lesions arising in the transverse and descending colon tend to be annular constrictive lesions, encircling the intestine and leading to obstruction. Sigmoid and rectal tumors may cause pressure on adjacent structures, such as the vagina, prostate, and bladder.

Symptoms of transverse/descending cancers:

- Change in bowel habits may become evident.
- Abdominal cramping, especially left lower quadrant pain.
- "Pencil" stools from narrowing of lumen. Constipation.
- Abdominal distension. Intestinal obstruction.
- Perforation of bowel/peritonitis.

Symptoms of sigmoid/rectal cancers:

- Tenesmus (painful, ineffective straining to pass stool).
- Pain in rectal or perianal area. Feeling of fullness and incomplete evacuation of stool after bowel movement.
- Alternating constipation and diarrhea.
- Frank blood in stool, possibly blood clots.
- "Pencil" thin stools from narrowing of lumen.
- Abdominal pain and cramping.
- Urinary symptoms.
- Vaginal fistula.

Neoadjuvant (Preoperative) Radiation and Chemotherapy

Advantages

A combination of radiation and chemotherapy given preoperatively has been shown to decrease the size of the tumor, allowing for more sphincter-saving procedures and a downstaging of the tumor grade. There is decreased seeding of the tumor in the operative site during surgery and less damage to the small intestine than is found with post-operative treatment. Reduction of the tumor results in better oxygenation to the surgical site. Studies have shown that neoadjuvant therapy is associated with a lower rate of metastasis and a higher rate of survival.

Disadvantages

The primary disadvantage to neoadjuvant therapy is an increase in the risk of post-operative complications, such as wound infections, bowel obstructions, fistulas, ischemic ileostomy and peristomal hernia. Additionally, because it is difficult to accurately stage a tumor prior to surgery, some people may receive treatment intended for a higher stage than their actual tumor. Over-treatment with chemotherapy and radiation therapy can have long-term side effects.

Crohn's Disease

Crohn's disease manifests with inflammation in any part of the GI system. Inflammation is transmural, often leading to intestinal stenosis and fistulas. Inflammation is focal and discontinuous with aphthous ulcerations that progress to linear and irregular shaped ulcerations. Granulomas may also be present. The most common sites of inflammation are the terminal ileum and cecum. Condition is usually chronic, but an acute flare-up may mimic appendicitis. Children may have delayed development and stunted growth. There appears to be a genetic component to the disease.

Symptoms include:

- Perirectal abscess/fistula may be present in advanced disease.
- Diarrhea is usually present with colonic disease. May have nocturnal bowel movements, watery stools, and rectal hemorrhage.
- Anemia may develop with chronic bleeding.
- Abdominal pain is most common in lower right quadrant, usually indicates transmural inflammation; may include post-prandial pain and cramping

Other symptoms include nausea and vomiting (usually related to strictures of small intestine), weight loss (with small intestine involvement), fever, and night sweats.

Ulcerative Colitis

Ulcerative colitis manifests with superficial inflammation of mucosa of colon and rectum, causing ulcerations in the areas where inflammation has destroyed cells. These ulcerations, ranging from pinpoint to extensive, may bleed and produce purulent material. The mucosa of the bowel becomes swollen, erythematous, and granular. Onset is usually between ages 15 and 30, and there is a genetic component. Ulcerative colitis may affect only the rectum (ulcerative proctitis), the entire colon (pancolitis), or only the left colon (limited or distal colitis).

Symptoms are as follows:

- Abdominal pain may be absent or mild unless disease is severe.
- Bloody diarrhea/rectal bleeding in absence of infection may result in anemia and loss of fluids and electrolytes. Diarrhea more frequent as colonic involvement increases.
- Fecal urgency and tenesmus (straining) may occur.
- Anorexia may result in weight loss, fatigue.
- Systemic disorders may manifest (eye inflammation, arthritis, liver disease, and osteoporosis) possibly because immune system triggers generalized inflammation.

Diagnostic Testing for Ulcerative Colitis and Crohn's Disease

Diagnostic testing for ulcerative colitis and Chron's disease includes:

- **Stool specimens** are examined for blood or pus or to rule out other disorders.
- **Flexible sigmoidoscopy** is useful for ulcerative colitis because the rectum is always affected. It can evaluate for mucosal inflammation, which is usually superficial.
- **Colonoscopy** shows extent of inflammation, especially for Crohn's disease.
- **Abdominal x-rays** can exclude complications.
- **Biopsy** shows tissue changes and lesions.
- **Technetium-labeled leukocyte scan** is used as less-invasive procedure for critically ill to determine extent of inflammation. It helps identify complications.
- **Complete blood testing** can show anemia, which may indicate chronic blood loss. Hypokalemia is related to chronic diarrhea. Hypoalbuminemia may reflect damage to mucosa of colon and/or malnutrition related to malabsorption.
- **Contrast radiography** with barium is useful for evaluating the upper GI tract for Crohn's disease.
- **CT scan, MRI, ultrasonography** may be used to identify complications
- **Serum anti-Saccharomyces cerevisiae antibody (ASCA) test** with positive finding is diagnostic of ulcerative colitis and indicative of Crohn's disease.

Diverticular Disease

Diagnostic Testing

Diverticular disease is the abnormal presence of sac-like pouchings in the intestinal lining. Diverticular disease is diagnosed by a number of tests, some used to rule out other disorders:

- **CBC and liver function tests** show white count is usually elevated, but liver enzymes remain normal.
- **Urinalysis** is usually normal with diverticular disease despite dysuria.
- **CT scan with contrast of abdomen** will show inflammatory changes and rule out other abdominal disorders.
- **Barium enema** may be used to show diverticula.
- **Ultrasound** uses high-frequency sound waves and a computer to create images of the soft tissue of the intestines. It may be used to rule out gall bladder disease or obstruction.
- **Colonoscopy/flexible sigmoidoscopy** can be used only when diverticulitis is NOT present to establish extent of disease. It is the most commonly used test for diverticular disease as it allows direct visualization as well as biopsy and surgical excision.

Risk Factors and Symptoms

Risk factors for diverticular disease include:

- **Age**: Incidence increases with age, affecting over 50% of those over 60.
- **Nationality**: More common in developed countries, such as the United States, England, and Australia where diets lower in fiber and high in processed carbohydrates are common. Diverticular disease is rare in Asian countries. People in Western countries primarily have diverticular disease in the left colon while Asians tend to have diverticular disease in the right colon.
- **Socioeconomic**: More common among those with lower income.
- **Genetics**: Occurs in family clusters.

Symptoms of diverticulosis (diverticula present but not inflamed):

- **Absent**: May have no symptoms at all.
- **Abdominal**: Cramping and distention.
- **Intestinal**: Constipation or diarrhea. Muscles spasms in colon.

Symptoms of diverticulitis (diverticula inflamed):

- **Systemic**: Fever, chills
- **Gastrointestinal**: Nausea, vomiting, constipation, GI bleeding, blood in stool, rectal bleeding.
- **Abdominal**: Mild to severe cramping, pain (especially in left lower quadrant), abdominal tenderness.
- **Urinary**: Dysuria may be present.

Neurogenic Bladder

Neurogenic bladder is bladder dysfunction from lesions of peripheral or central nervous system, related to traumatic or congenital etiologies or develop from cerebrovascular accident or diabetic neuropathy. Nerve damage can cause underactive bladder unable to contract to effectively empty the bladder or overactive bladder that contracts frequently and ineffectually. **Symptoms** vary:

- **Underactive**: Incontinence, dribbling, straining or inability to urinate, retention.
- **Overactive**: Frequency, urgency, dysuria, urinary tract infection, fever.

Diagnosis is by:

- **Neurological testing (x-rays, MRI, and EEGs)**: To determine etiology. 24-hour urine collection: To determine volume and urine patterns.
- **Bladder stress test**: To determine reaction to full bladder while bending over, coughing, walking, or doing other activities.

Treatment includes:

- **Antibiotics**: To control infections.
- **Clean intermittent catheterization** (CIC): To empty bladder.
- **Endoscopy**: Combined with cutting of external sphincter or injecting sphincter with paralytic agents to allow urination.
- **Surgical repair**: Placing of permanent stents at bladder neck, bladder augmentation to increase bladder size, repair of vesicoureteral reflux, or urinary diversion.

Diagnostic Testing for Radiation Enteritis, Ischemic Colitis, Intestinal Obstruction, and Gastrointestinal Trauma

Radiation enteritis:

- **Endoscopy** is used to examine intestinal mucosa for changes consistent with radiation enteritis.

Infectious enteritis:

- **Stool specimens** are examined for occult blood, ova and parasites, other organisms, and white blood cells to determine infecting agent.
- **Endoscopy** provides direct examination of the lumen of the intestines.
- **Biopsy** is done for tissue analysis and culture to identify the infecting agent.

Intestinal obstruction:

- **CT scan of abdomen** helps identify causes and location of obstruction.
- **Complete blood testing** helps to eliminate infections and other diagnoses.
- **Laparoscopy** allows direct visualization of obstruction to determine best procedure for correction.

Intestinal trauma: Tests relate to severity and location of trauma and may include a wide range, including.

- **CT scan** is done to determine the extent of the injury and complications.
- **Complete blood testing** is done to determine blood loss, clotting times, and oxygen saturation.

Hirschsprung's Disease

Hirschsprung's disease is a congenital disorder in which infants are born without intestinal ganglion nerve cells in part or the entire colon, causing mechanical obstruction. It may be an acute life-threatening or chronic condition.

Normally, nerves signal the colon to contract, pushing the stool through the colon, but the absence of propulsion in the segments without ganglions causes the fecal material to accumulate. Affected areas almost always include the rectum and distal colon, but in rare instances can skip segments and involve the entire colon, including the small intestine. As fecal material collects, the segment of the bowel proximal to the defect distends, creating megacolon. The internal rectal sphincter may fail to relax as well, preventing evacuation and contributing to obstruction. Hirschsprung's disease accounts for about 25% of all neonatal obstructions, is 4 times more common in males than females, may have a genetic link, and is more common in children with Down syndrome.

The **symptoms** of Hirschsprung's disease in the neonatal period, infancy, and childhood are as follows:

- Neonatal period:
  - No meconium within 24-48 hours after birth, although rectal stimulation during the physical exam after birth may cause a small amount of meconium to be expelled.
  - Reluctance to nurse/bottle feed. Vomitus stained with bile. Abdominal distension from gas and accumulated fecal material.

- Infancy:
  - Underweight/failure to thrive. Chronic constipation.
  - Abdominal distension. Episodes of diarrhea and vomiting.
  - Loud bowel sounds with gurgling. Enterocolitis—fever, explosive watery diarrhea (stool frothy, green with foul odor), severe prostration with symptoms of sepsis.
- Childhood:
  - Thin, poorly nourished appearance. Anemia. Chronic cycles of constipation. Foul stools with ribbon-like appearance.
  - Abdominal distension with visible peristaltic waves. Fecal masses palpable in abdomen.

Diagnosis is based on symptoms, which may vary, so diagnosis may be delayed until infancy or childhood when acute enterocolitis occurs. Procedures include:

- Abdominal x-rays. Barium enema done without preparation.
- Anorectal manometry. Full-thickness rectal biopsy showing absence of ganglion cells.

Imperforate Anus

Imperforate anus (anorectal malfunction) is a congenital abnormality where the rectum is absent, malformed, or displaced from normal position. It may include disorders of the urinary tract. Imperforate anus occurs in 1 in 5000 births, more commonly in males than females. Imperforate anus may include stenosis or atresia of anus. There are 3 main categories, classified according to relationship of rectum to puborectalis musculature:

- **Low anomalies**: No external opening, but rectum is otherwise in normal position through the puborectalis muscle, with normal function, and no connection to the genitourinary tract.
- **Intermediate anomalies**: Rectum is at or below the level of puborectalis muscle and an anal dimple is evident. The external sphincter is in normal position.
- **High anomalies**: Rectum ends above the puborectalis muscles, and internal sphincter is absent. Frequently, there is a rectourethral fistula in males or a rectovaginal fistula in females. There may be fistulas to the bladder or perineum.

Symptoms include:

- **Absence of anal opening**: No meconium in 24-48 hours, Abdominal distension, and vomiting.
- **Rectovaginal fistula or rectourethral fistula**: Symptoms may not be evident at first because stool passes through fistula.
- **Fistula between the rectum and the bladder**: Gas or fecal material may be expelled per the urethra.
- **Displacement of the anus**: Chronic constipation develops over time.

Diagnosis includes:

- Physical examination.
- Digital or endoscopic examination.
- Contrast radiography with the infant inverted and an opaque marker at the anal dimple will outline the location of a pouch in relation to the normal position of the anus.

Most forms of **treatment** require surgery, type depending upon extent of abnormality:

- Simple excision for anal opening may suffice.
- 2-3 step procedures for higher anomalies in which a colostomy is first performed with later reconstruction of the anus in the proper position, involving anoplasty and pull through procedures.
- Manual dilation may treat stenosis.

Necrotizing Enterocolitis

Necrotizing enterocolitis is acute inflammatory disease of bowel, especially in preterm and high-risk infants, resulting in necrosis and frequent perforation, affecting large or small intestines or both and often the ileocecal area. "Skip" areas of necrosis may be present, making surgical treatment difficult. The causes of necrotizing enterocolitis are not completely clear, but vascular compromise occurs, often related to an episode of hypoxia or sepsis or post blood transfusion. The hypoxic condition in the intestines causes damage and necrosis to mucosal cells so bowels can't secrete protective mucus, making the intestine susceptible to bacterial infection. Three factors are implicated: feeding, injury to intestinal mucosa, and bacterial infection.

Symptoms usually appear 3-10 days after childbirth and range from mild Abdominal distension to severe sepsis:

- Hypotension.
- Apnea.
- Decrease in urinary output.
- Vomiting/gastric retention.
- Temperature fluctuations.
- Irritability.
- Lethargy.
- Blood in stools or gastric aspirate (occult or gross).
- Poor feeding.

Diagnosis includes:

- **Careful physical examination**: Observing for signs of peritonitis
- **Monitoring of abdominal girth** to determine degree of distention.
- **Laboratory findings**: Neutropenia, thrombocytopenia, and metabolic acidosis. Abdominal x-rays: One every 6-8 hours to observe for perforation. Contrast studies: Carry risk of perforation, but are occasionally done with water-soluble contrast medium.

Treatment:

Both **medical** management and **surgical** repair may be needed although severely compromised infants are not good surgical candidates:

- **Medical treatment**: Discontinuation of oral fluids and administration of intravenous fluids. Nasogastric decompression. Correction of fluid and electrolyte imbalances. Oxygen to correct hypoxia. Systemic antibiotics for infection. Transfusions.

- **Surgical treatment**: Varies, depending upon extent and location of necrosis, and may involve creation of ileostomy, jejunostomy, or colostomy as permanent or temporary diversion. Some surgeons remove clearly necrotic tissue while others avoid resection. One or more stomas may be established. Closure of stoma is usually done 1-4 months after initial surgery.

Malrotation and Omphalocele

Malrotation is an abnormality during fetal development in the rotation and fixation of the midgut area. With ischemia or bowel necrosis, pre- or post-operatively, fecal diversions may be needed.

Omphalocele is a congenital herniation of intestines or other organs through the base of the umbilicus with a protecting amniotic membrane but no skin. The sac may contain only a loop or most of the bowel and the internal abdominal organs. This sac differentiates gastroschisis from omphalocele. Diagnosis is usually with fetal ultrasound.

Symptoms vary widely. Maintaining integrity of tissues by keeping exposed sac or viscera moist and providing intravenous fluids is important. Small omphaloceles are repaired immediately, but more extensive repair is usually delayed until the infant is stable if the sac is intact. Silvadene® cream toughens the sac, which is usually covered with a Silastic® (plastic) pouch to protect the tissue. The abdomen may be unusually small, making correction difficult, so surgeons may wait 6-12 months while the abdominal cavity grows. Surgical repair may be done in stages over 8-10 days.

Gastroschisis

Gastroschisis is extrusion of the non-rotated midgut through the abdominal wall to the right of the umbilicus with no protective membrane covering matted, thickened loops of intestine. The abnormality is usually small, but the stomach and almost all of the small and large intestines can protrude. Because the intestines float without protection in amniotic fluid, there may be severe damage to the intestines with bowel atresia and ischemia. Gastroschisis is usually diagnosed with fetal ultrasound and is obvious at birth. These infants lose body temperature, fluids, and electrolytes and receive intravenous fluids. The exposed organs are covered with sterile plastic film for protection and to prevent fluid loss and a nasogastric feeding tube is inserted. Primary closure is done when the infant stabilizes for small abnormalities. Larger abnormalities may require stages with only part of organs returned to the cavity and the remaining covered with a Silastic pouch until the abdominal cavity grows and surgical repair can be completed.

Umbilical Hernia

An umbilical hernia is a skin-covered herniation of intestine and omentum through an abdominal wall defect near the umbilicus caused by an incomplete closure of the umbilical ring. The herniation may range from 1-5 cm in size and may be obvious on physical examination or felt on palpation. It may appear flat when the child is supine but protrude when the child is upright or crying. Approximately 1 in 6 infants are born with umbilical hernias. Symptoms are usually absent unless strangulation of the hernia occurs, and then the infant may cry with pain, feed poorly, vomit, and have an increase in temperature. The abdomen may become distended. In this case, emergency surgical repair must be done. Treatment usually involves just observing the hernia for complications as, in most cases it will reduce on its own. If the hernia is still present at 3-4 years, a simple surgical repair of the hernia may be done.

Mesocolic Paraduodenal Hernia

Mesocolic paraduodenal hernia is an internal herniation of the small intestinal loops in the paraduodenal area due to incomplete rotation of the small intestine, resulting in intestinal loops becoming trapped in the mesentery of the descending colon. Right and left hernias are separate entities. Right (Waldeyer's hernia) results in the small bowel being trapped behind the mesentery of the right and transverse colon. With left, the herniated sac is to the left of the duodenum and the inferior mesenteric vessels are on the anterior margin. Some infants are asymptomatic and the condition may go undiagnosed. Infants may have frequent indigestion, and some go on to develop chronic digestive problems, but acute bowel obstruction with strangulation and perforation may occur. Radiographic studies with contrast are done for diagnosis. Surgical reduction with repositioning of the bowel is done to repair the hernia if there are no complications, such as strangulation, which may require more extensive repair.

Congenital Diaphragmatic Hernia

Congenital diaphragmatic hernia is herniation of abdominal contents into chest cavity. During fetal development, a hole in the diaphragm that should close at about 3 months stays open, allowing loops of the intestine or the stomach to herniate into the chest and preventing adequate development of the lungs (pulmonary hypoplasia) and/or heart. The infants are usually very dyspneic at birth and may need to be ventilated. They may need temporary heart/bypass as well. The kidneys are often enlarged. Radiographic studies are done to show the extent of the abnormality, usually showing a high gastrointestinal obstruction, often at the duodenum. A nasogastric feeding tube is inserted and an intravenous line. Supportive treatment is given for dyspnea as well as correction of acidosis. Surgical repair may be done after birth or delayed for weeks until child stabilizes. Surgical repair may be done in one stage or more, depending upon the degree of abnormality.

Intussusception

Intussusception is telescoping of one portion of intestine into the next, usually distal small intestine near ileocecal junction moving into the ascending colon and causing obstruction, inflammation, edema, and ischemia of the involved intestine. It usually occurs between 5-10 months, but can occur from 3 months to 6 years. It occurs 3-4 times more frequently in males.

Symptoms include:

- Acute onset of severe intermittent abdominal pain.
- Loud frantic crying with knees drawn to chest.
- Vomiting.
- Bloody mucoid stool resembling currant jelly.
- Sausage-like abdominal mass, usually in right upper lateral region and along transverse colon.

Diagnosis is by physical examination, abdominal x-rays or ultrasound, and contrast enemas.

Treatment includes:

- **Non-surgical**: Hydrostatic reduction using barium or air if no evidence of peritonitis or gangrene.
- **Surgical**:
    - Laparotomy with manual reduction.
    - Resection and anastomosis: Irreducible areas dissected.
    - Fecal diversion (rare): If bowel ends too inflamed and swollen for anastomosis.

Meconium Ileus

Meconium ileus is the obstruction of the ileum with inspissated (thick) mucilaginous meconium that clings to the side of the narrowed lumen of the intestine and forms hard pellets in infants with cystic fibrosis. This is usually the first clinical sign of cystic fibrosis. A complicated meconium ileus may involve volvulus, gangrene, perforations, peritonitis, or bowel atresia. Meconium ileus must be differentiated from Hirschsprung's disease, which presents with similar symptoms.

Symptoms include:

- **Uncomplicated**: Abdominal distension, vomiting, no meconium in first 24-48 hours.
- **Complicated**: Pain, fever, erythema, and edema of abdominal wall consistent with peritonitis.

Diagnosis is by abdominal x-rays to show air-fluid levels and contrast enemas to show obstruction.

Treatment:

Contrast enema with water-soluble contrast: May relieve obstruction by emulsifying fecal material. 10-15 cc small volume enemas: To flush stool, especially after contrast enema. Enterotomy: With proximal instillation of wetting agent. Resection of colon/fecal diversion: For perforated or gangrenous bowel.

Persistent Cloaca

Persistent cloaca is a condition in females with an **imperforate anus** and the rectum, vagina, and urethra forming a **single channel**, with a rectal fistula attached to the posterior wall of the channel. Diagnosis is made with a physical exam showing a single perineal opening. An abdominal mass (hydrocolpos— distended bladder) may occur. A voiding cystourethrogram (VCUG) will show bladder abnormalities if catheterization is possible.

Treatments include:

- **Colostomy**: Fecal diversion in neonate prevents fecal material from entering urinary system and causing infection.
- **Decompression of vagina**: Decompression prevents infection and scarring and relieves obstruction of urinary tract.
- **Posterior sagittal anorectovagino-urethroplasty (PSARVUP)**: This is usually done 2 months after colostomy. The rectum is separated from the vagina, the vagina is separated from the urethra, the urethra is reconstructed, the vagina is reconstructed, and the rectum is reconstructed with anoplasty.
- **Postoperative anal dilation**: Dilation begins 2 weeks after surgery until final size is reached.
- **Cystoscopy/ vaginoscopy**: Check for urethrovaginal fistula.
- **Colostomy removal**: Anastomosis of colon and rectum and colostomy removed.

Cloacal Exstrophy

Cloacal exstrophy is a rare and complicated disorder of pelvic area, usually including multiple abnormalities, such as omphalocele with abdominal viscera covered by thin membrane outside of abdomen; exstrophy of bladder, which is bivalve and surrounds the intestinal mucosa at midline and communicates with the rectum; imperforate anus; spinal defects; and genital abnormalities, such as vaginal duplication, agenesis, or atresia. May also include multiple urinary, spinal, and skeletal abnormalities. **Symptoms** vary widely depending on abnormalities. **Diagnosis** is made by physical examination and renal ultrasound to assess kidneys.

Treatment:

Surgical repair is done in stages, beginning with separation of urinary and intestinal systems and creation of intestinal stoma. If possible, primary closure of bladder and repair of omphalocele are done with initial surgery. Reconstruction of urinary and reproductive system is usually done when the child stabilizes and weight is ≥9 kilograms. The intestinal stoma is permanent, but urinary continence may be through urinary diversion or reconstruction.

Bladder Exstrophy

Bladder exstrophy is eversion of posterior wall of the bladder through anterior wall of the bladder and through the lower abdominal wall with bladder and urethra exposed, a wide pubic arch, anterior displacement of the anus, renal disorders, and abnormalities of reproductive organs in both males and females. **Symptoms** include urinary and bowel problems related to specific anomalies. **Diagnosis** is by physical examination to assess abnormalities. Renal ultrasound is done to determine the number of kidneys and presence of hydroureteronephrosis.

First stage treatment includes:

- **Primary closure of bladder**: No ostomy necessary if done within 72 hours of birth. Procedures include ureteral stents and suprapubic urinary drainage.
- **Bilateral iliac ostomies**: Necessary after 72 hours because pelvic ring is not malleable.
- **Epispadias repair**: May be done in first or second stage.

Second stage treatment includes:

- **Epispadias repair**: Usually done between 6-12 months.

Final stage of treatment includes:

- Bladder neck reconstruction and reimplantation of ureters.
- Permanent urinary diversion: Required by 10-15%.

Megaureter

Megaureter is dilation of ureters from the normal 3-5 mm to more than 10 mm in diameter with or without obstruction and/or reflux from abnormality of ureters or secondary causes:

- **Primary obstruction**: At point where ureter joins bladder; can cause kidney damage.
- **Refluxing**: Backward flow of urine from bladder to ureters.
- **Non-obstructing/non-refluxing**: Dilated ureters without blockage may resolve over time.
- **Obstructed/refluxing**: Ureters continue to dilate with blockage.
- **Secondary**: Ureters enlarge because of other conditions, such as neurogenic bladder.

Symptoms include urinary tract infection, dysuria, back pain, and fever.

Diagnosis is by:

- **Fetal ultrasound**: in utero diagnosis
- **Ultrasound**: To evaluate appearance of urinary tract
- **Voiding cystourethrogram (VCUG)**: To check for reflux
- **Diuretic renal scan**: To check for obstruction
- **Intravenous pyelogram**: To view urinary system

Treatment includes:

- **Antibiotic prophylaxis**: Until surgery.
- **Ureteral implantation**: Trimming widened portion of ureter; removing obstruction and reattaching.

Prune Belly (Eagle-Barrett) Syndrome

Prune belly (Eagle-Barrett) syndrome is a group of abnormalities involving lack of developed abdominal muscles, undescended testicles, and urinary tract problems. Urinary abnormalities may include large, hypotonic bladder, dilated ureters, and prostatic urethra. Males comprise 96-99% of cases. It may include anomalies of the pulmonary, cardiac, skeletal, and GI tracts.

Symptoms vary widely, frequently including cardio-pulmonary complications:

- **Prune-like appearance of abdomen**: From fetal Abdominal distension. After birth, abdominal fluid is lost and abdomen develops wrinkled "prune" appearance, noticeable because of undeveloped abdominal muscles. Undescended testicles: Bilaterally.
- **Urinary tract abnormalities**: Urinary infections, obstruction, and chronic renal failure. Diagnosis is by physical examination, chest x-rays to evaluate pulmonary problems, renal ultrasound to evaluate kidneys, and voiding cystourethrogram (VCUG) to evaluate urinary defects.

Management includes the following:

- Monitor condition. Antibiotics, therapeutic and prophylactic.
- Intermittent catheterization. Surgical repair to correct genitourinary defects varies according to abnormality. Procedures may include: Vesicostomy, ureterostomy, or pyelostomy.
- Reduction cystoplasty, urethroplasty.
- Abdominoplasty.

Ureteropelvic Junction Obstruction

Ureteropelvic junction obstruction (UPJ) is congenital obstruction at the point where the ureter connects to the renal pelvis, unilaterally or bilaterally, causing inadequate urinary flow and hydronephrosis. Some children improve markedly within the first 18 months, but others require surgery.

Symptoms include:

- Urinary tract infections.
- Abdominal or flank pain
- Palpable mass from hydronephrosis.
- Vomiting.

Diagnosis is based on:

- **Fetal ultrasound**: in utero diagnosis.
- **Renal ultrasound**: To show dilation of renal pelvis.
- **Intravenous pyelogram (IVP)**: To identify obstruction.
- **Renal isotope scan**: To evaluate and measure kidney function.

Treatment includes:

- **Fetal urinary diversion**: Remains controversial.
- **Pyeloplasty**: Open surgical procedure where ureteropelvic junction is excised and ureter reattached to renal pelvis with wide junction, allowing adequate drainage.
- **Laparoscopic pyeloplasty**: Through abdominal wall and abdominal cavity with internal excision of ureteropelvic junction.
- **Insertion of wire through ureter**: To cut ureteropelvic junction from inside with a ureteral drain left in place for a few weeks.

Vesicoureteral Reflux

Vesicoureteral reflux is an abnormality where urine flows from the bladder back up the ureter. Reflux is graded on a scale of 1-5, depending upon the degree of dilation of the ureter and renal pelvis.

- **Primary**: Congenital defect with impaired valve where ureter opens to bladder. The ureter may be too short so the valve doesn't close properly.
- **Secondary**: Caused by infection or other cause of obstruction.

Symptoms of urinary tract infection are most common:

- **Neonates**: Fever, irritability, lethargy, emesis.
- **Older infants, children**: Abdominal pain, emesis, diarrhea, fever, dysuria with enuresis, frequency, urgency, cloudy/foul urine.
- **Late symptoms**: Hypertension, dysuria with difficulty urinating, proteinuria, chronic renal insufficiency.

Diagnosis is by:

- **Ultrasound**: Evaluate appearance of urinary system.
- **Voiding cystourethrogram (VCUG)**: Identify reflux (after infection has cleared).
- **Intravenous pyelogram**: Reveal obstructions.
- **Nuclear scans**: Show urinary functioning
- **Cystoscopy**: View bladder interior.

Treatment includes:

- **Antibiotics**: For infection.
- **Surgical repair/reconstruction**: Usually involves severing ureter from bladder and reattaching at a different angle to prevent reflux.

Epispadias and Hypospadias

Epispadias is a condition in which the urethral orifice is in an abnormal position with a widened pubic bone. In boys, the urethra may open on the top (dorsum), the sides, or the complete length of the penis. In girls, the urethra, with a urethral cleft along its length, usually bifurcates the clitoris and labia but may be in the abdomen. Boys may have a short, wide penis with abnormal chordee (curvature). Epispadias is 3-5 times more common in males than females. Hypospadias, which occurs only in males, is a condition in which the urethral orifice opens onto the ventral surface of the penis.

Diagnosis is by physical exam and endoscopy to evaluate bladder neck and external sphincter. Intravenous pyelogram evaluates the urinary tract.

Symptoms for both conditions include urinary incontinence, infections, and reflux nephropathy (backward flow of urine to kidneys). **Treatment** is surgical repair to lengthen the urethra (and penis, in males) and reconstruct the bladder neck. Multiple surgical procedures may be required for both males and females. Urinary diversion may be necessary if incontinence cannot be corrected.

Myelomeningocele with Lipoma and Tethered Cord

Myelomeningocele is meninges and spinal cord herniating (neural tube defect) through bony defect in the vertebra (spina bifida) anterior or posterior, with protrusion usually in the lower back, with or without lipomas (fatty lesions that grow around the spinal cord) and/or tethered cord (fatty tissue at base of spinal cord that "tethers" the vertebra, stretching it as the child grows). May also have scoliosis, kyphosis, or lordosis.

Symptoms include:

- **Hydrocephalus**: Affects about 30%.
- **Urinary incontinence**: Most have constant leakage of urine but may not empty bladder completely. Others have detrusor-sphincter dyssynergia (sphincter fails to relax).
- **Neurogenic bowels**: Chronic constipation with altered sensation and sphincter control, fecal incontinence.

Diagnosis is by physical exam with posterior lesions evident and MRI for diagnosis of anterior lesions, lipomas, and tethered cord.

Treatment includes:

- **Surgical repair** of neural tube defect/Ventricular-peritoneal shunt.
- **Urinary care**: Clean intermittent catheterization (CIC).
- **Vesicostomy/continent urinary diversion**: To manage incontinence.
- **Bowel management**: Diet and habit training.
- **Appendicostomy**: To allow easy irrigation of bowel.

Posterior Urethral Valves

Posterior urethral valves (PUV) are a urethral abnormality in males where urethral valves have narrow slit-like openings that impede urinary flow and allow reverse flow, damaging urinary organs, which swell and become engorged with urine. Thirty percent with PUV will develop long-term kidney failure. **Symptoms** vary depending upon severity:

- **Dysuria**: Pain, weak stream, frequency.
- Hematuria. Urinary retention. Incontinence. Enlarged bladder palpable as abdominal mass. Urinary infection (most common symptom after 1 year of age). Sepsis, metabolic acidosis, and azotemia (increased blood levels of urea and other nitrogenous compounds) may develop.

Diagnosis consists of the following:

- Fetal ultrasound.
- Voiding cystourethrogram (VCUG): Evaluate extent of valvular abnormality and other urinary defects.
- Endoscopy: Examine inside of urinary tract/take tissue samples. Blood tests: Assess kidney function and electrolytes.

Treatment includes:

- Supportive care, antibiotics, electrolytes, Foley catheter.
- Urinary diversion: Usually closed after valve repair.
- Endoscopic ablation/resection: Examine obstruction and remove valve leaflets.

Hereditary Non-Polyposis Colorectal Cancer (HNPCC)

HNPCC is an inherited autosomal-dominant syndrome where people develop a few polyps and cancer at about age 40. Two clinical variants exist:

- **Lynch I** is early onset of cancer, usually in proximal bowel.
- **Lynch II** is nonpolyposis colon cancer with cancer of endometrium, ovary, small bowel, and urinary tract.

There are **two criteria for genetic testing**:

- **Amsterdam** determines if family members need testing. At least 3 relatives (2 first degree) in 2 successive generations have colorectal cancer, one before 50.
- **Bethesda**—one of following criteria means the person with colorectal cancer should have cancer cells checked for microsatellite instability (MSI)—changes in DNA of cells, giving rise to mutations:
    - Colorectal cancer before 50.
    - History of another cancer associated with HNPCC.
    - History before 60 of cancer with characteristics of MSI.
    - First-degree relative before 50 has non-colorectal cancer often found in HNPCC carriers.
    - Two or more second-degree relatives have HNPCC-related tumor at any age.

Familial Adenomatous Polyposis (FAP)

FAP is an inherited autosomal-dominant syndrome where people develop hundreds to thousands of colorectal polyps between ages 5-40 with cancer usually in one or multiple polyps by about age 20. Between 20-40, virtually everyone develops cancer. A genetic factor predisposes people with this genetic mutation to other malignancies, especially in duodenum and stomach. They may develop Gardner syndrome with congenital hypertrophy of retinal pigment (CHRP), sebaceous cysts, desmoid tumors (fibrous tumors arising in tissue covering intestines), and benign bone tumors. Identifying FAP before colorectal cancer develops is critical as prophylactic colectomy may be indicated with high risk. People with familial history of FAP should have genetic testing.

Variant forms of FAP:

- **Attenuated familial adenomatous polyposis** has delayed polyp growth, with onset of colorectal cancer at about 55 years of age.
- **Autosomal recessive familial adenomatous polyposis** typically causes fewer than 100 polyps and is caused by mutation on different gene than other forms.

Anorectal Fistulas (Fistula-In-Ano)

Anorectal fistulas are those extending from the anal canal to the perineal skin. Most anorectal fistulas originate in the anal glands, which are located between the layers of the anal sphincters and drain into the anal canal. If the glands become blocked and an abscess forms, it can begin to tunnel toward the surface of the skin. There may be only one tunnel or tract, but there may also be multiple. Abscesses can become recurrent if they heal over at the surface. As purulent material collects beneath the healed surface, pressure builds, and it breaks through again. Anorectal fistulas are common in those with Crohn's disease and can occur with rectal cancer or after radiation.

Symptoms include:

- Swelling, pain, and discharge (purulent or sanguinous).
- Diarrhea.
- Anal bleeding.
- External opening of fistula.

Treatment includes:

- **Antibiotics**: To treat infection/abscesses.
- **Seton**: Suture holding fistula opening (draining seton).
- **Fistulotomy/fistulectomy**: Excision (most effective but contraindicated with Crohn's disease.)

ENTEROCUTANEOUS FISTULAS

Enterocutaneous fistulas are those extending from the intestine to the skin. The most frequent causes are Crohn's disease, cancer, anastomotic leak, bowel obstruction, and sepsis. They may develop post-operatively or spontaneously. If excess pressure develops on an anastomosis, a fistula can develop. Malignancy, infection, steroids, and poor nutrition are all contributing factors. Fistulas seek weakness in tissues and thus may exit through wounds, incisions, drain sites or compromised tissue.

Symptoms include:

- **Local**: Erythema, evident opening, purulent/sanguinous discharge.
- **Systemic**: Sepsis, fever, electrolyte imbalance, anemia, malnutrition, dehydration.

Treatment includes:

- **Decrease secretions**: Restrict fluids, Somatostatin to decrease small bowel secretions.
- **Nutritional support**: Enteral (if only colon affected) or total parenteral support.
- **Surgery**: Surgical closure may be done if spontaneous closure unlikely. Usually delayed for 6 to 8 weeks after sepsis controlled to allow for spontaneous closure if possible and reduce the risk of peritonitis. May be done in stages for complex fistulas.

COMMON CAUSES OF FISTULAS

Common causes of fistulas include:

- **Intestinal diseases**: Inflammatory bowel disorders such as ulcerative colitis and Crohn's disease as well as diverticulitis are associated with inflammation, infection, and ulceration, leading to formation of fistulas.
- **Cancer**: Rectum, colon, bladder, or any cancer in the abdomen or pelvic area can cause trauma that result in fistulas.
- **Abscess**: About 50% of abscesses develop fistulas, regardless of the cause of the abscess, so they are always a cause for concern.
- **Surgery**: Any surgery involving the pelvic organs or the intestines can result in fistulas, especially with infections and abscess formation. Cholecystectomy is a common cause of fistula formation.
- **Radiation**: Pelvic radiation, especially, is a common cause of vesicovaginal fistulas.
- **Trauma**: Fistulas are a possibility with many types of traumatic injuries. Trauma from obstructed labor during childbirth is a frequent cause of vesicovaginal and rectovaginal fistulas. Rape, especially gang rape, has been implicated as a frequent cause of fistulas.

Obtaining the Health History

Interview Process

The nurse should review previous medical records and have a clear idea of the purpose of the **interview** and should outline questions. If possible, the patient should be interviewed alone or should be asked if he/she wants family members present. Both verbal and nonverbal responses should be observed during an interview. Important factors include:

- **Initial introductions**: Make introductions by name and explain roles and the purpose of the interview, asking how the patient wishes to be addressed and avoiding using familiar terms, such as "dear," which may be considered condescending. Stress the confidential nature of the interview and explain who will receive the information.
- **Interview structure**: The interview may be somewhat unstructured, guided by patient responses, or may be very structured with the nurse asking a list of questions, but the nurse must remain flexible while still guiding the discussion in order to accommodate different communication styles.
- **Appearance**: The nurse should be professionally dressed and wearing a clear nametag. The patient's appearance should be observed non-judgmentally for clothes (loose/tight clothes may indicate weight change), cleanliness (dirty clothes/skin/hair may indicate cognitive or physical impairment or poverty), and demeanor (calm, fidgeting, nervous).

Initial Assessment of Patient Requiring Fecal and/or Urinary Diversion

History and presentation: The initial assessment will focus on everything that has led the patient to needing a fecal and/or urinary diversion. This can include other treatments that have been utilized if there is a chronic disease involved, or the details of an acute event or trauma that has occurred.

Comorbidities: Any other disease states that may affect the patient's ability to recuperate from the surgery should be considered. This can include cardiovascular disease or diabetes. Chronic conditions that may impair a patient's ability for self-care are also important considerations.

Age: The impact of having a permanent fecal or urinary diversion can vary at different points in a person's life. Young patients that are otherwise healthy may have a different prognosis than elderly patients with comorbidities. Age may also obstruct the ability to self-care or retain education received regarding the fecal/urinary diversion.

Medications: Reviewing all medications that a patient is taking before surgery is important. For example, a patient who is taking medication for Crohn's disease may not require this after a fecal diversion is placed. Depending on the location of the diversion and the type of medication, absorption rates may be affected. It is important for the patient to review all medications with their provider or pharmacist prior to surgery.

Psychological issues: The stress of undergoing surgery, along with the impact the diversion will have on the patient's life, should be considered. Any issues of depression or anxiety should be addressed with appropriate referral to a mental health professional if necessary.

Interpreting Lab Values for Ostomy Patient

Hemoglobin – Carries oxygen and is decreased in anemia and increased in polycythemia. Used to assess bleeding. Normal values:

- Males >18 years: 14.0-17.46 g/dL.
- Females >18 years: 12.0-16.0 g/dL.

Hematocrit – Indicates the proportion of RBCs in a liter of blood (usually about 3 times the hemoglobin number). Used to assess bleeding. Normal values:

- Males >18 years: 45-52%.
- Females >18 years: 36-48%

Glucose – High levels are indicative of diabetes, which predisposes to skin injuries, slow healing, and infection:

- Normal values: 70-99 mg/dL.
- Impaired: 100-125 mg/dL.
- Diabetes: ≥126 mg/dL.

Serum creatinine – Increases with impaired renal function, urinary tract obstruction, and nephritis. Level should remain stable with normal functioning.

- Normal values: 0.6-1.2 mg/dL.

Blood urea nitrogen (BUN) – Increase indicates impaired renal function, as urea is end product of protein metabolism.

- Normal values: 7-8 mg/dL (8-20 mg/dL >age 60).

White blood cell (leukocyte) count is used as an indicator of bacterial and viral infection. WBC is reported as the total number of all white blood cells.

- Normal WBC for adults: 4,800-10,000.
- Acute infection: 10,000+; 30,000 indicates a severe infection.
- Viral infection: 4,000 and below.

The differential provides the percentage of each different type of leukocyte. An increase in the white blood cell count is usually related to an increase in one type, and often an increase in immature neutrophils (bands), referred to as a "shift to the left," is an indication of an infectious process:

- Normal immature neutrophils (bands): 1-3%. Increase with infection.
- Normal segmented neutrophils (segs) for adults: 50-62%. Increase with acute, localized, or systemic bacterial infections.
- Normal eosinophils: 0-3%. Decrease with stress and acute infection.
- Normal basophils: 0-1%. Decrease during acute stage of infection.
- Normal lymphocytes; 25-40%. Increase in some viral and bacterial infections.
- Normal monocytes: 3-7%. Increase during recovery stage of acute infection.

Medical Treatments for Urinary Incontinence

Medications for urinary incontinence:

- **Antispasmodics (tolterodine, oxybutynin, hyoscyamine)**: for overactive bladders. These drugs may cause thirst, so longer-acting preparations of these drugs, which have fewer side effects, may be better for some people.
- **Antidepressant (imipramine)**: to relax the bladder and contract the muscles at the bladder neck:
- **Hormone replacement therapy**: Administered as a vaginal cream, ring, or patch to protect bladder and urethral mucosa. Oral estrogen may not be as effective as topical for incontinence.
- **Antibiotics**: To treat infections that may be causing or worsening incontinence.
- Some medications, such as sedatives, may increase or cause incontinence, so all medications should be assessed.

Medical devices:

- **Catheters**: Clean intermittent catheterization to empty bladder.
- **Penile clamps**: Apply pressure around the penis to clamp the urethra.
- **Pessaries**: A stiff ring inserted vaginally to treat bladder prolapse.
- **Urethral inserts**: Urethral inserts may be inserted temporarily during times of activity that may prompt incontinence.

Foods That Can Cause or Relieve Problems with Ostomies After Bowel Surgery

Foods that may cause obstruction include:

- **Fruits**: Dried fruits, fruits with seeds (such as pomegranates and figs) and skin (such as cherries), large servings of raw fruit.
- **Nuts**: Tree nuts (such as walnuts and almonds), peanuts, and popcorn.
- **Vegetables**: Whole corn, bean sprouts, bamboo shoots, large servings of raw vegetables, celery, mushrooms.

Foods that may cause diarrhea/loosening of stool include:

- **Fruits**: Juices (especially apple and prune juice), prunes, fresh fruit.
- **Vegetables**: Broccoli, cabbage, raw vegetables.
- **Other**: Spicy foods, fried foods, baked beans, sugar-free gum.

Foods that may cause constipation/thickening of stool include:

- **Fruits**: Applesauce, bananas.
- **Proteins**: Cheese, creamy peanut butter.
- **Starches**: Potatoes (without skins), rice, pasta, whole wheat bread, tapioca pudding, marshmallows.

Foods that may cause gas/odor include:

- **Vegetables**: Cabbage, broccoli, kale, cauliflower, kohlrabi, Brussels sprouts, asparagus, onions, dried peas, rutabagas, and turnips.
- **Proteins**: Dried beans fish, strong cheeses, and eggs.
- **Other**: Spicy foods, chewing gum.
- **Drinks**: Beer, carbonated beverages (such as sodas or juices).

Diet and Fluid Modifications

After Continent Cutaneous Fecal Diversions and Ileal Pouch Anal Anastomosis

After continent cutaneous fecal diversions (continent ileostomy) and ileal pouch anal anastomosis, the pouch will stretch and consistency of stool will thicken in the months following. Monitoring diet and fluids can control bowel movements and prevent dehydration. Meal times may need to be adjusted for better control, especially at night.

- **Eat**: Regular meals are important. After surgery, eating helps to stretch the pouch and food will slow down the frequency of bowel movements. Gas forms when bowels are empty, so eat small frequent meals.
- **Add foods**: Try one new food at a time to determine tolerance. Many people are lactose intolerance, so be careful with dairy products. Cheese can help to slow stools.
- **Starch**: Rice, potatoes, and pasta once a day can help to slow stools.
- **Potassium**: Foods high in potassium, such as bananas and potatoes, can help to prevent hypokalemia from diarrhea.
- **Simple sugars**: Can cause diarrhea, so limit.
- **Fluids**: Drink 6 to 8 glasses of fluid a day, but not with meals.

People with Continent Cutaneous Urinary Diversions

For individuals with **continent cutaneous urinary diversions**, it is important to maintain adequate kidney function by drinking 8-10 glasses of fluid daily. The pH of the urine ranges normally from 4.6-8, in the acidic range and an effort should be made to maintain acidity. Alkaline urine is more likely to become infected and develop crystals. Most meats and cereals produce acidic urine, but most fruits and vegetables produce alkaline urine.

- **Odor-producing foods**: Fish, asparagus.
- **Acid foods**: Grains and cereals, meats, cheese, corn, crackers, cranberries, eggs, pasta, nuts, rice, prunes, plums, fish, and poultry.
- **Alkaline foods**: Bananas, beans, beets, milk, greens, most fruits (including citrus fruits such as oranges and lemons), most vegetables.

Including acid foods as part of daily diet and making some substitutions, such as drinking cranberry juice instead of orange juice, can help to keep the urine acidic. Taking daily vitamin C, with permission of physician, can also help to keep the urine acidic.

Environmental, Social, and Other Factors That Impact Patient's Adaptation

Environmental factors such as living alone or being homeless can add to the burden. Lacking a support system or having non-supportive family and friends may increase fear and depression.

Social factors such as low income or lack of insurance make the cost of colostomy supplies prohibitive.

Cultural factors also have an impact. Mexican families are often patriarchal with the eldest male in the family consulted first. Asians often believe people should not receive bad news about their health and may want to keep diagnostic information secret. Religion is also a consideration. Muslims may be concerned about the gender of healthcare providers. Jews, Hindus, and Muslims may want the body to remain intact. Hindus and Buddhists may believe their condition is related to karma. Folk beliefs must be respected and an attempt made to integrate into plan for care.

Other factors include **language barriers**. A translator and the use of teaching materials in other languages may be required.

Psychosocial Factors Affecting Care

Psychosocial factors affecting care include:

- **Ability to learn/perform care**: Cognitive impairment and hearing or vision deficits may interfere with the ability to learn, especially if appropriate educational materials are not available. Physical disabilities may make it difficult to patients to learn or perform some aspects of care. Language differences may result in impaired comprehension.
- **Economic implications**: Patients and families may be severely impacted if the wage earner is unable to continue to work or if they lack the resources (insurance, financial) to pay for needed care.
- **Education**: Patients may lack an adequate educational background to understand the implications of disease, to read materials, and to follow directions. Health literacy may be very low, so patients may have misconceptions about disease.
- **Mental status**: Patients often experience increased stress associated with illness, and this may interfere with functioning. Mental impairment may impact ability to participate in care. Additionally, depression is common, especially with chronic illness, and may cause patients to withdraw or fail to comply with treatment.

Coping Strategies for Fecal or Urinary Incontinence While in Social Situations

The following are coping strategies that people with fecal or urinary incontinence can use to manage when they are outside of the home in social situations:

- Plan:
    - Schedule activities, if possible, at times with less chance of fecal/urinary incontinence. Use the toilet before leaving home.
    - Wear an incontinence pad or disposable underwear as needed.
    - Wear clothing that is comfortable and not constricting.
    - Carry pre-moistened wipes, extra pads, ostomy supplies as needed. Keep extra clothes, supplies/disposable underwear somewhere that is easily accessible.
- Survey environment:
    - Locate the bathrooms before an urgent need arises so they can be accessed easily.
    - If more than one bathroom is available, determine which provides the most privacy.
- Practice prevention:
    - Sit so exit to the bathroom is convenient, at end of a row or table rather than in the middle.
    - Use toilet periodically at whatever schedule gives best control, probably at least every 2 hours.
    - Avoid foods or drinks, such as carbonated beverages, that may cause gas or stimulate bowels/bladder. Foods to avoid are often individual based on experience.

Surgical Indications and Procedures

Surgery for Colorectal Cancer

Indications for colorectal surgery include:

- **Prophylactic**: To prevent cancer, often for precancerous polyps.
- **Diagnostic**: Biopsy to confirm diagnosis and determine type of cancer. Various surgical techniques may be used.
- **Staging**: To determine extent of malignant invasion. Surgical staging is more accurate than imaging or laboratory findings.
- **Curative**: Removal of tumor to affect a cure. It is considered the primary treatment but may be done in conjunction with chemotherapy or radiotherapy.
- **Cytoreductive**: Debulking removes all possible tumors without damaging organs or surrounding areas and may be done when it's impossible or too dangerous to remove entire tumor. It may be followed by chemotherapy or radiotherapy.
- **Palliative**: To alleviate symptoms or discomfort; not curative.
- **Supportive**: To assist with other treatments. May include installation of catheter port into large vein for delivery of chemotherapy or blood testing.
- **Restorative**: To restore function, as when colostomy is removed and bowel reattached.

Surgical Options for Hirschsprung's Disease

Surgical treatment for Hirschsprung's disease used to always be done in two stages, with a temporary colostomy performed proximal to the aganglionic segment to allow the bowel to heal and regain tone prior to the final surgical procedure. However, earlier diagnosis has resulted in most children having one-step procedures. All procedures are pull-through in that the aganglionic portion is removed and the functioning portion of bowel is "pulled through" and attached to the anus:

- **Swenson procedure**: This procedure retains a small 1-2 cm section of aganglionic sleeve through which the functioning bowel is pulled through and sutured to the anus.
- **Duhamel procedure**: This procedure uses a stapler to connect aganglionic segment to functioning bowel so that the aganglionic segment constitutes the anterior wall but the posterior wall has enervation.
- **Soave procedure**: This procedure brings the functioning bowel down through the sleeve of the rectum where it is attached to the anus.

Surgical Treatments for Urinary Incontinence

There are over 200 different surgical procedures to treat disorders that cause incontinence. Common options include:

- **Artificial urinary sphincter**: Fluid-filled ring placed around bladder neck to keep the sphincter closed. A valve under the skin is pushed to deflate the ring to allow urination. Procedure is rarely done on women.
- **Augmentation cystoplasty**: A section of the colon is removed, shaped, and sutured into the bladder wall to expand the bladder capacity.
- **Injections of bulking agents**: Collagen is injected to the tissue around the urethra or urinary sphincter to tighten the sphincter for women. Must be repeated every 6-18 months.
- **Sacral nerve stimulation**: Small device is implanted in the abdomen with a wire to the sacral nerve to stimulate the bladder.

- **Sling procedure**: Abdominal, donor, or synthetic tissue placed under the urethra, acting like a hammock and compressing urethra to prevent leakage for women.
- **Urinary diversion**: Cystectomy with urinary diversion as last resort for intractable incontinence.

Indications for Fecal Diversion Surgery

Indications for fecal diversion surgery are as follows:

- Inflammatory bowel disease:
  - **Crohn's disease** may affect any part of the GI system, especially the ileum. It may cause swelling and lesions that involve all layers of the intestinal wall.
  - **Ulcerative Colitis** causes inflammation and ulceration of the large intestine, but only in the top layer of the intestinal wall.
- Gastrointestinal cancers:
  - Rectal or colon cancer may metastasize or obstruct.
  - Rectal obstruction may result from metastasis of advanced pelvic cancer
- Gastrointestinal and non-gastrointestinal etiologies:
  - **Diverticular disease** with complications may result in abscess, obstruction, fistula or perforation of intestine. Radiation enteritis may cause malfunction from intestinal damage. Ischemic colitis most often of the left colon may cause irreversible damage.
  - **Infectious enteritis** may be caused by bacteria, viruses, parasites, or fungi. Hospital stay and/or antibiotic use may lead to Clostridioides difficile infection, which may lead to severe complications. Intestinal obstruction, mechanical or non-mechanical, can lead to necrosis. Gastrointestinal trauma related to blunt or penetrating injuries may damage part of intestine.

Indications for Urinary Diversion Surgery

Bladder cancer with cystectomy results from either primary bladder cancer or cancer originating in pelvic organs. Bladder cancer may result from chronic irritation caused by indwelling catheters or when bladders are left intact after urinary diversion surgery.

Prostate cancer may advance to cause ureteral obstruction from lymph node involvement or from invasion of the base of the bladder.

Neurogenic bladder, bladder dysfunction from lesions of the peripheral or central nervous system, may be related to traumatic or congenital etiologies. It may also develop after cerebrovascular accident or from diabetic neuropathy.

Interstitial cystitis causes chronic debilitating pain of the bladder, urethra, and pelvic area as well as dysuria. It may relate to congenital or traumatic injuries that cause inflammation and problems with urine storage and bladder emptying. Pain may persist after surgery.

Refractory radiation cystitis is damage caused from radiation treatments, resulting in intractable incontinence or urinary fistulas.

Procedures for Hartman's Pouch and Colonic J Pouch

Hartman's pouch: To create a Hartman's pouch, the intestine is severed, usually with removal of a part of the distal segment because of a cancerous lesion. The proximal end is brought through the abdominal wall to form a stoma for fecal drainage. The non-functioning distal end of the colon with the rectum intact is stapled or stitched to close and then left in place, forming a non-functioning pouch.

Colonic J pouch: To create a colonic J pouch requires a two-step procedure. In the first step, a temporary loop ileostomy is performed for fecal diversion above the surgical site, and a newly constructed pouch from a 6-10 cm segment of colon is attached to the rectal stump after removal of a cancerous lesion, creating the J pouch. In the second step, after about 2-3 months, the ileostomy is reversed and anastomosis is done to re-establish intestinal continuity.

Operative Procedures for Rectal Cancers/Colostomies

Abdominal peritoneal resection: The rectum, anus, and sphincter are removed and the distal end of the sigmoid colon is used to form a stoma in the left lower quadrant. Used commonly for low rectal cancers.

Coloanal anastomosis: This sphincter-preserving procedure entails removal of cancerous bowel proximal to the rectum and then anastomosis of the distal end of the remaining colon to the rectum, above the levator ani muscles, leaving a 1-2 cm distal margin. Best for women with gynecoid pelvis and people who are not obese and lack complications or pre-surgical fecal incontinence.

Low anterior resection: The lower rectum is left intact and an anastomosis is done below the peritoneal reflection. Used for cancers in the upper and middle thirds of the rectum.

Combined low anterior resection with coloanal anastomosis: This combination procedure is usually done with anastomosis completed after temporary fecal diversion gives tissue time to heal.

Colostomy Irrigation

The following considerations should be made as it relates to colostomy irrigation:

- **Type of colostomy**: People who had regular bowel habits before surgery and have permanent colostomies in the descending or sigmoid colon are good candidates for irrigation because the stool is usually formed rather than liquid at this part of the colon.
- **Contraindications**: People with prolapse or hernia should not irrigate as the irrigation may worsen the conditions.
- **Motivation**: Irrigation requires people to be committed to and be physically able to perform the procedure by themselves or with the assistance of caregivers on a regularly scheduled basis.
- **Constipation**: Since constipation and impaction can still occur, this must be managed as well by medications, such as stool softeners, or diet, fluid, and exercise. Irrigation can help relieve chronic constipation.
- **Regulation**: Irrigation is usually done every 1-2 days. Once the ostomy is regulated, without fecal leakage between irrigations, a stoma cap can be used between irrigations rather than a pouch.

Low Anterior Resection (LAR)

Low anterior resection is a sphincter-sparing procedure for rectal cancer (stage I, II, or III) occurring in the anterior portion of the rectum. LAR may be done as an open surgical procedure or through a minimally invasive laparoscopic procedure with site election guided by ultrasound and MRI. LAR involves removing the rectum (completely or partially) about the lesion and lymph nodes and then attaching the remaining rectal tissue to the colon. The procedure avoids creation of a permanent colostomy although some patients may require a temporary ileostomy to allow the tissue to adequately heal, especially those who have undergone radiotherapy and/or chemotherapy. However, complications may occur and may impair the quality of life. LAR syndrome, which occurs when the anal sphincter is injured or innervation impaired, may result in chronic leakage of fecal material, urgency, frequent bowel movements, constipation, or impaction. These symptoms may persist for years or become permanent. Treatment includes Kegel exercises, medications (loperamide, psyllium), biofeedback, stool training, and emotional support.

Total Proctocolectomy

A total proctocolectomy is removal of the entire rectum, colon, and anus through an open surgical procedure or minimally-invasive laparoscopic procedure. Total proctocolectomy may be done for cancer, severe inflammatory bowel disease (Crohn's disease, ulcerative colitis), toxic megacolon, uncontrolled GI bleeding, or intestinal perforation. Total proctocolectomy requires an alternate method of fecal evacuation, so this may involve creation of an ileostomy or, in some cases, a J pouch. If the total proctocolectomy is combined with an ileostomy, the ileostomy is created during the initial surgical procedure. However, if a J-pouch is constructed (most common for ulcerative colitis), two or three stages are utilized. In the first stage, the rectum is retained but is later removed and the J-pouch created along with a temporary loop ileostomy to allow the J-pouch to heal. Complications of total proctocolectomy may include postoperative ileus, infection, hemorrhage, necrosis, intestinal obstruction, and sepsis. With a pouch, pouchitis, and pouch-anal/vaginal fistulae may also occur.

Continent Cutaneous Fecal Diversion (Continent Ileostomy)

Continent ileostomy: May be done after proctocolectomy; the lower part of the small bowel is used to create an internal reservoir for collection of fecal material. This pouch is created from the small intestine and has a leak-free nipple valve inside the abdominal stoma, also created from the intestine to prevent leakage of stool, with an intestinal conduit leading to the pouch.

This type of pouch is a **Kock pouch**, named after the physician who developed the procedure. The valve-modified T-pouch or Barnett pouch is also sometimes used. It is usually done for either ulcerative colitis or familial adenomatous polyposis (FAP). Pouch is emptied 4 times daily through a plastic catheter. The continent ileostomy has been superseded by newer techniques, such as the restorative proctocolectomy with the J pouch, but it is still useful for those over 50, those who are incontinent, or those whose J pouches have failed.

Intubation and Dressing Supplies for Continent Cutaneous Fecal Diversions

Choice of supplies depends on personal preference as well as factors such as mucus production or leakage of stool:

- **Intubation supplies**: Most people use a 30-34 Fr. catheter to drain continent ileostomies. There are a number of brand names, such as Marlen, Medina, Weber and Judd and Mentor. Some have a bullet tip with holes on the side. Others have a rounded tip with a hole at the tip and on the side. Some catheters are straight, and others are curved, but all are flexible. If straight catheters are stored coiled for a length of time, they tend to stay curved. They range from 12-18 inches in length and can be trimmed to preferred length.
- **Dressing supplies**:
    - Absorbent pads with hypoallergenic adhesives, often 4x4.
    - Stoma caps in various shapes and sizes, look like flesh-colored adhesive bandages.
    - Nursing pads/eye pads are inexpensive, easily available substitutions for stoma dressings.

Ileal Pouch Anal Anastomosis (IPAA)

Ileal Pouch Anal Anastomosis: Involves leaving rectal sphincter intact with excision of colon and creation of temporary ileostomy. A reservoir (pouch) is constructed of small intestine pulled down and sewn or stapled to the anal muscles.

- Ileo-anal pull-through: Distal end of small intestine is pulled through rectal stump and sutured to the anus.
- The J, S, and W (named because of the appearance of the looped intestines) pouches are made by looping the intestine side-by-side, detubularizing, and then suturing together to make a larger pouch.
    - J Pouch—2 limbs of small intestine are used to create a pouch.
    - S Pouch—3 limbs are used.
    - W Pouch—4 limbs are used.

The ileostomy is taken down after about 2 months, giving the pouch the time to heal. The reservoir capacity will be small at first with 10-12 stools per day, but the pouch will stretch and frequency will decrease to 4-5 stools per day.

Detubularization

Detubularization refers to the preparation that takes place to prepare an intestinal segment for use in the construction of a urinary reservoir. The intestinal segment is divided and then sewn back together to create a spherical rather than tubular reservoir. Intestinal segments have a muscular layer which contracts to carry out peristalsis and propel the fecal material through the intestines. When a segment of the intestine is removed and attached elsewhere in the body, the intact tubular intestine retains the ability to contract, and this would apply too much pressure within the reservoir and prevent adequate stretching. To accommodate this intestinal characteristic, the tubular intestinal segment is opened lengthwise along the anti-mesenteric border to reduce or eliminate muscle tone. It is sutured together again in such a way as to interfere with peristaltic activity. This effectively decreases the pressure generated by the newly-formed reservoir and increases its capacity.

Orthotopic Neobladder

Orthotopic neobladder is the creation of a reservoir to serve as a urinary bladder in the normal bladder position. The bladder is usually removed, and a urinary reservoir is made out of segments of the ileum or colon, including the ileocecal valve. The long intestinal segment, usually from the ileum, is detubularized before being shaped into a pouch. The ureters are attached superiorly in a refluxing manner. Sometimes, the ureters may be anastomosed to a short limb of the small bowel, a configuration known as the Studer pouch, and allowing easy conversion of neobladder to an ileal conduit if necessary. The urethra is anastomosed to the reservoir. During surgery, a urethral catheter is placed to drain urine and perform as a stent. There are ureteral catheters and often a suprapubic catheter and drains in place as well; all drains except for Foley catheter are usually removed before discharge. Foley remains about 3 weeks.

Surgical Placement Methods for Gastrostomy Tubes

Gastrostomy is a permanent or temporary opening into the stomach. While percutaneous endoscopic gastrostomy is standard for feeding tubes, with hypopharyngeal or esophageal carcinomas, stenosis may prevent oral feeding and endoscopy, so surgical methods are used.

- **Janeway** is a laparoscopic procedure where the gastric mucosa is sutured/stapled to the abdomen, creating a permanent continent gastrostoma in the left upper quadrant through which intermittent catheterization provides long-term feeding.
- **Stamm** is an open procedure where a midline incision opens to the anterior aspect of the stomach with a stab incision into which a balloon catheter is inserted with purse-string sutures to tighten the opening around the catheter. The stomach wall is sutured to the anterior abdominal wall at the exit site, providing a secure opening for catheters.
- **Witzel** is an open procedure where a serosal tunnel of tissue in the gastric wall covers 4-6 cms on the implanted tube, making a permanent tract and securing the tube.

Placement for Gastrointestinal Feeding Tubes

The three types of placement for gastrointestinal feeding tubes are summarized below:

- **Surgical placement**: There are both open and laparoscopic surgical techniques for tubes to the stomach or jejunum. The three most common methods are the Janeway, the Stamm, and the Witzel techniques.
- **Endoscopic placement**: Percutaneous endoscopic gastrostomy (PEG) involves intubation of the esophagus with the endoscope and insertion of a sheathed needle with a guidewire through the abdomen and stomach wall so that a catheter can be fed down the esophagus, snared, and pulled out through the opening where the needle was inserted and secured. Similar endoscopic procedures can be done in the jejunum.
- **Radiologic placement**: Through fluoroscopy, ultrasound and/or CT, gastrostomy tube is inserted through the epigastrium and secured with a balloon and external bumper or disk. Insertion into the jejunum is done in a similar manner through the duodenum into the jejunum. A gastrojejunostomy tube, which both drains the stomach and feeds the jejunum, is another procedure.

Surgical Jejunostomy for Feeding Tubes

Jejunostomy: Creation of an opening into the jejunum beyond the ligament of Treitz for insertion of feeding tube.

- **Indications**: This procedure is indicated for those with high risk of aspiration (such as those with neurologic disease or decreased awareness), esophageal or gastric cancer, oropharyngeal dysmotility, or previous surgery of stomach, duodenum, or pancreas. Those suffering from dysphagia should be evaluated as potential candidates for jejunostomy rather than gastrostomy. Jejunostomy decreases the risk of aspiration pneumonia.
- **Procedures**: Open surgical or laparoscopic techniques may be used to create the jejunostomy. Both the Stamm and the Witzel procedures that are used for gastrostomy may be modified to use with jejunostomy. With the Stamm procedure, the jejunum is secured to the abdominal wall to make a secure opening for the balloon feeding tube. With the Witzel procedure, a seromyotomy creates a tunnel by involuting the jejunal wall over the tube.

Bolus/Syringe, Gravity Drip, and Pump Feedings Per Enteral Tubes

Feeding tubes should be checked and flushed before infusion. The type and amount of feeding solution is prescribed by physician.

- **Bolus/syringe feedings** use a 60-cc catheter tip syringe attached to the end of the feeding tube. The tube is clamped until the formula is poured into the syringe, unclamped, and the formula allowed to flow in by gravity. Raising or lowering the syringe will speed or slow flow.
- **Gravity drip feedings** use a feeding bag filled with formula from the top. The measures are marked on the outside to help monitor inflow. Roller clamps control the rate of flow. Feedings may be continuous or for a prescribed number of hours. The bag should be changed at least every 24 hours to prevent bacteria from growing.
- **Pump feedings** use an electrical or battery-powered device to control rate of infusion when the tubing is fed through the device, allowing precise control of the infusion rate.

Insertion of Balloon Replacement Gastrostomy Tube

Insertion of a balloon replacement gastrostomy tube:

1. Gather supplies, position patient to 30 degrees, wash hands.
2. Inject 20 mL sterile water into balloon port to check balloon leaks. Withdraw water and retain filled syringe.
3. Apply gloves and move external disk to near distal end.
4. Lubricate catheter tip with water-based lubricant.
5. Cleanse peristomal area with normal saline in spiral movement. Dry skin.
6. Insert tube gently to pre-measured distance. Do not force. Turn tube if resistance met or withdraw and try different angle until in place. (If unable to insert, call physician.)
7. Inflate balloon through balloon port, using correct amount of water.
8. Gently pull tube until resistance met. Slide external bumper to 1.5 cm from skin surface.
9. Rotate tube in circular motion to ensure free rotation.
10. Use 30-60 mL syringe to aspirate gastric content. Flush tube with water.
11. Clean skin, apply barriers as needed, and mark exit measurement with tape flag or indelible ink.

Removal of Balloon Replacement Gastrostomy Tube

Removal procedure:

1. Gather the supplies for a clean procedure. Sterile gloves are not necessary.
2. Reassure patient that the procedure is not painful and explain the steps. If reinsertion is to be done, explain that procedure as well.
3. Position patient's head no higher than 30 degrees.
4. Wash hands.
5. Schedule removal for 2 hours after continuous feeding or prior to bolus feeding so residual feeding solution doesn't drain onto the skin as this could cause irritation.
6. Using a 20 mL Luer-Lok syringe inserted into the balloon port, slowly deflate the internal balloon.
7. Measure extracted fluid to make sure the balloon is completely deflated, and then gently pull the tube out. If resistance is met, rotate tube and try again.
8. Cover stoma with gauze pad until reinsertion of new tube. Reinsertion should immediately follow removal of tube to prevent tract closure.

Managing Fecal/Urinary Diversions in Special Populations

Neonatal

Education will be geared toward the parents/caregivers of the infant. With fecal diversions, a pouch that will accommodate increased gas should be used. Any changes in the stoma size should be regularly assessed, also, as this will change the barrier and pouch sizes as the infant grows.

Pediatric

Once a child reaches 5 or 6 years of age, they can usually start learning how to care for a diversion. Size and fit should be considered, especially as the child begins to be more active. Issues with body image will begin as the child matures.

Adolescent

Body image issues are a major concern at this age as the adolescent patient matures and lives with a fecal or urinary diversion. The patient can learn how to care for the diversion on their own. Support groups consisting of other adolescents with fecal/urinary diversions can be very helpful at this age, when social acceptance is a priority.

Bariatric

Body habitus can affect the stoma size and location. Larger patients with multiple skin folds can increase the risk of skin breakdown or skin infection. If morbidly obese, there may also be issues of the patient performing self-care of the diversion.

Assessing Ability to Provide Self-Care

A number of issues are important when assessing the patient's ability to provide self-care:

- **Manual dexterity**: Both fine and gross manual dexterity should be assessed to determine the patient's ability to carry out any necessary treatment and to perform procedures. Additionally, the patient's manual dexterity may impact the person's ability to perform ADLs. Testing may include asking patients to pick up small items with tweezers, place pins in a pegboard, grasp, lift, and throw.
- **Vision**: The patient should wear glasses when vision is assessed. Impaired vision can impact the patient's ability to safely take medications, carry out ADLs, and do treatments. Testing may include asking the patient to read and to describe something at a distance.
- **Cognition**: Impaired cognition may interfere with all aspects of self-care. If a patient has mild cognitive impairment, instructions may need to be broken down into very simple steps, but with more severe impairment, the patient may need assistance. Testing may include questions (name, birthdate, residence, date), simple memory tasks (remember 3 items after a few minutes), drawing (face of a clock), and talk back (asking patient to demonstrate or explain to show understanding).

Focused Assessment of Urinary and Fecal Diversions

Continent Cutaneous Urinary Diversion

Continent urinary diversion: Involves construction of a urinary reservoir to which ureters are attached. The reservoir has some type of valve inside the stoma to prevent leakage. There are a number of different types of pouches, which are modifications of the original Kock pouch, which has 3 segments: a nipple made by intussuscepting 17 cm of small bowel to form a 5 cm segment. A second small intestinal segment is used to create a stoma in the abdominal wall. The third segment is a 78 cm segment that is looped into a u-shape, opened, and sutured together to create a U-shaped pouch to which the ureters are implanted. The ureters also have valves to prevent backflow.

Other pouch techniques: Several pouches involve the use of part of the right colon as well as the small intestine: Indiana, Florida, Miami, and Mainz pouches. The Florida pouch has consistently the highest degree of continence.

Urostomy

A urostomy is a procedure by which urine is redirected to a stoma in the abdominal wall. This type of urinary diversion drains urine constantly and requires the use of a pouch.

There are **two main types of urostomies**:

- **Ileal conduit**: This is the oldest urinary diversion procedure and has few complications. In this procedure, about a 12 cm loop of ileum (or in some cases colon) is cut from the intestine and the intestine is then reconnected. One end of this intestinal "tube" is sutured to the abdominal wall to create a stoma and the ureters are attached to the other end, thus creating an ileal conduit for urinary flow. Stents are usually placed in the ureters to maintain patency.
- **Ureterostomy**: This procedure is rarely done now except as a temporary measure in pediatric patients. In this procedure, the ureters are directly connected to the abdomen, creating one or two small bud stomas.

Colostomy

A colostomy is the general term that involves removal of part of the colon with the end of the remaining colon sutured to the abdominal wall to create a stoma, or opening, through which stool can pass.

The following are terms related to colostomies:

- **Permanent**: A permanent colostomy is usually done after part of the colon, usually the rectum and lower colon, is excised without plans for reanastomosis.
- **Temporary**: A temporary colostomy allows the part of the colon distal to the stoma to rest or heal until the two parts of the colon can be reattached or reconstruction completed.
- **End**: An end colostomy is a temporary (as above) procedure or a permanent procedure where a stoma is created proximal to an inoperable carcinoma to allow for fecal diversion and to prolong life.
- **Ascending**: An ascending colostomy creates a stoma from the ascending portion of the colon on the right side of the abdomen.
- **Descending/sigmoid colostomy**: The descending or sigmoid colostomy is the most common type and creates a stoma from the end of the sigmoid (descending) colon, usually in the lower left abdomen.

- **Loop**: A loop colostomy creates one stoma with two openings, one for stool and the other for mucus, usually in the transverse colon. May have a supporting rod in place. This is a common procedure for short-term fecal diversion.
- **Transverse**: The transverse colostomy creates one or two stomas from the transverse colon, usually in the upper abdomen in the middle or on the right side.
- **End-loop**: Loop of intestine is brought to abdominal wall with both proximal and distal end stomas side by side. Often used as a temporary procedure for obstructed colon.
- **Hidden colostomy**: A loop of intestine is retained in subcutaneous fat and left for easy access in case a colostomy becomes necessary at a later date.

Ileostomy

The following are the two main types of ileostomy:

- **End (standard, Brooke's)**: The end of the ileum is brought up through the abdominal wall to create a stoma, usually after the colon and rectum are surgically removed. If some colon and the rectum remain but are sutured closed and left below the surface, this type of ileostomy is a temporary procedure. The stoma is usually small and round and fairly easy to pouch.
- **Loop**: A loop of the ileum is brought through the abdominal wall. A rod may be placed beneath the loop to keep it elevated above the skin. The loop is opened to allow for fecal drainage from the proximal portion of the loop and mucus from the distal portion. The loop is usually temporary, allowing the colon to heal, and this construction allows for easy closure of the ileostomy. Loop ileostomies tend to have larger misshapen stomas that are more difficult to pouch.

Absorption Concerns for Medications for Those with Continent Cutaneous Fecal Diversions

Because of the loss of the colon and less time in the intestine, enteric-coated medications or time-release capsules may not be absorbed completely or at all. Uncoated tablets or liquid medications usually are absorbed; however, if the food is passing through the ileostomy undigested, there may be decreased absorption of even these medication forms.

- **Antacids**: Magnesium can cause diarrhea.
- **Antibiotics**: May cause diarrhea and dehydration.
- **Antidiabetics**: Glucophage may not be absorbed properly.
- **Birth control pills**: May not be completely absorbed, making them unreliable.
- **Corticosteroids**: Can cause sodium retention and fungal infection under faceplate of pouch because of suppression of immune system.
- **Diuretics**: May cause electrolyte imbalance.
- **Laxatives**: Should NOT be taken. Can cause electrolyte imbalance.
- **NSAIDs**: May cause gastric bleeding or duodenal-gastric irritation. Take with food.
- **Sulfa drugs**: Usually cause no problem.
- **Vitamins**: Liquid form is absorbed best. Vit B-12 should be given by injection or nasal spray.

Fecal Diversion Pouchitis

Pouchitis is a non-specific inflammation of the mucosal lining of the internal (ileo-anal, Kock, J, W, S) pouch created from part of the small intestine after colectomy. It usually occurs during the first two years after surgery. It is most common among those with ulcerative colitis, affecting 20-30%.

About 5-7% of those with pouchitis will have chronic recurring episodes. Pouchitis rarely requires removal of the pouch. Acute episodes last fewer than 4 weeks; chronic, more than 4 weeks.

Symptoms include:

- **Stools**: A steady increase in the frequency of stools is the most common problem. The person affected may also develop incontinence of stools, watery, or bloody stools. A feeling of urgency is also common.
- **Pain**: May have crampy abdominal pain.
- **Systemic**: Fever, dehydration from excessive loss of fluids.

Treatment includes:

- **Antibiotics**: 1-2 weeks course of metronidazole or ciprofloxacin.
- **Probiotics**: Replacement of normal intestinal flora.
- **Steroids**: Oral and topical, including budesonide.
- **Immunosuppressives**: Infliximab.

Dehydration, Hyponatremia, and Hypokalemia

Electrolyte imbalance, especially loss of potassium and sodium, poses a problem for people with the large intestine removed. Any increase in fluid loss, such as diarrhea, perspiration, or vomiting, can exacerbate the imbalance. Generally, avoidance of a low salt diet and salting to taste helps to maintain sodium levels.

Dehydration:

- **Symptoms**: Thirst, dry mouth, loss of skin turgor, decreased urinary output, headache, lethargy, abdominal cramping.
- **Treatment**: Increase fluid intake to 8-10 glasses daily and include fluids high in electrolytes, like Gatorade.

Hyponatremia:

- **Symptoms**: Anorexia, headaches, drowsiness, cramping of legs and abdomen, dizziness, postural hypotension, arms, and legs feel cold.
- **Treatment**: Increase intake of high sodium foods and fluids, like canned soup, bouillon, ham, Gatorade, soy sauce, buttermilk.

Hypokalemia:

- **Symptoms**: weakness in muscles, fatigue, gas, Abdominal distension, shortness of breath, decrease in sensation of arms and legs.
- **Treatment**: Increase intake of orange juice, bananas, chicken, fish, pinto beans, potatoes, raisins, tomatoes, watermelon, yogurt, and Gatorade.

Stoma Complications

Assessment for Stomal and Peristomal Complications

Stoma assessment includes the following:

- **Type** of stoma may be fecal or urinary and constructed from small intestine, colon, bladder, or ureters. Diversion may be continent or incontinent.
- **Characteristics** of stoma include moist mucosa. Color depends on tissue used in construction. Stoma from intestines is red and beefy looking; from ureter or bladder, pale pink.
- **Edema** is usually present, so stoma should be measured routinely to determine changes.
- **Shape and size** may vary depending upon surgical technique and effects of peristalsis. Some are round; others, oval.
- **Protrusion** of stoma should be slightly above skin to provide for proper pouching, but stomas may retract below the skin or prolapse.
- **Function** depends upon type of ostomy and position. Urostomies produce urine immediately, but colostomies may not excrete stool for 4-5 days and ileostomies, 24-48 hours.
- **Peristomal skin** should be clear of irritation and intact with intact suture line.

Ostomy Signs and Symptoms That Require Follow-Up Care

Ostomy signs/symptoms requiring follow up care include:

- **Changes in functioning**: Any change in the normal function of an ostomy (constipation or diarrhea, change in character of stool/urine) or indications of blockage are a concern.
- **Changes in appearance**: The stoma, peristomal area, and any surgical incisions should be monitored carefully for changes. If the stoma becomes dusky, edematous, depressed, or prolapsed, this needs attention. The peristomal area should remain clear of any irritation.
- **Increase in pain**: Pain should decrease in the post-operative period, but if there is an increase in pain, especially with sudden onset, this could indicate an infection, obstruction, or other complications that need immediate attention.
- **Bloody or purulent discharge**: Stomas, peristomal areas, and discharge should be examined for signs of bleeding or infection. Any indication of blood or pus in feces or urine should be cause for concern.
- **Abdominal distension**: An increase in Abdominal distension, especially if accompanied by other symptoms such as pain or bleeding, may indicate complications.

Stomal Complications

Ischemia/Necrosis

Ischemia/necrosis is a lack of circulation resulting in cyanosis and discoloration of the stoma, from dark red to blue to black. Ischemia may occur within a few hours of surgery or up to 5 days postoperatively. It may be the result of too much mesenteric tension compromising circulation, which can result from edema, obesity, distention of the abdomen. It can also result from an embolism that impairs circulation. As condition worsens, it may be complicated by **mucocutaneous separation.** Sutures that are too constrictive have also been implicated. If necrosis is superficial, it may heal as necrotic tissue sloughs. However, with deeper necrosis or profound circulatory impairment, surgical repair is usually necessary to prevent infection or perforation. It's important to use clear pouches that are properly fitted after surgery so that ongoing assessment of the mucosa can be done in order to prevent deep necrosis and resulting complications.

Ileus

Ileus is the lack of intestinal contractions and bowel sounds because of paralysis of the bowel caused by excessive manipulation during surgery, prolonged period of anesthesia, or narcotic pain medications. This can result in a non-functioning stoma, as the fecal material remains trapped. Individuals should be encouraged to exercise and roll from side to side frequently to stimulate contractions. Ileus may require nasogastric tube to decompress the stomach and prevent vomiting until normal bowel activity returns.

Peristomal Abscess

Peristomal abscesses are characterized by open lesions that are painful with surrounding erythema. They are common when there is active Crohn's disease in the section of the bowel distant to the stoma. The abscess may need to be opened by the surgeon to promote drainage. Treatment will vary depending upon size and degree. Hydrophilic or hydrocolloid materials may be used as a barrier. A non-adhesive pouching system may be used during the healing process.

Prolapse

Prolapse is telescoping of the bowel 5 or more inches with mucosal edema, related to large fascial opening in abdominal wall, colostomy through abdominal incision, or obstruction at surgery. A pouching system should be used to accommodate the prolapse at its largest size, and pouches with rigid rings should be avoided. The person should be taught techniques to reduce the prolapse, such as lying flat, applying pressure/ice pack. The person should be taught signs of ischemia.

Hemorrhage

Hemorrhage is active bleeding with considerable blood loss and is usually caused by an open mesenteric vessel. Superficial bleeding may be the result of trauma to the stoma and is usually self-limited. Heavy bleeding may relate to underlying liver disease. Bleeding may result from anticoagulant therapy or steroids as well. Identifying the cause of the bleeding is critical for treatment. Pressure should be applied to control bleeding, but surgical repair may be necessary to stop bleeding.

Mucocutaneous Separation

Mucocutaneous separation is separation of the stoma from the skin at the suture line as a result of inadequate healing, increased tension, or infection. If the separation is superficial, it may be easily treated, but deeper separations pose a more difficult management problem. Additionally, the separation may be in just one area or completely around the stoma. Mucocutaneous separation is treated conservatively to allow healing unless there is a danger of contamination of the peritoneum that may result in peritonitis. In that case, the area may be resutured. For small open areas, skin barrier powder, hydrofiber, or calcium alginate can be used as absorbent material to fill open space, and appliance should be fit over this barrier. Rope packing may be used for deeper separations. If there is considerable drainage, this open draining area may need to be pouched with the stoma to prevent peristomal irritation.

Retraction

Retraction occurs when the stoma pulls below the skin level, caused by tension below the stoma from a variety of factors, including excessive scar formation, obesity, inadequate stoma length, recurrence of active Crohn's disease, and improper excision of skin. Management includes using a convex pouching system with a belt. Surgical revision may be needed.

Stenosis

Stenosis is contraction and narrowing of the stoma, resulting from ischemia. A low residue diet, increased fluids, and stool softeners may prevent blockage. Stoma dilation may be used or surgical revision.

Trauma

Trauma is injury to the stoma mucosa usually related to pouch injury or pressure from a hard surface, such as a belt or tight clothing rubbing up against the stoma or constricting it. It is important to determine the cause of the trauma and to correct this so that it does recur. In severe cases of trauma, a transparent pouching system should be used until healing to allow visualization of the stomal circulation.

Fistula

Fistula is an abnormal opening between the stoma and the skin. It is usually related to recurrence of disease after an ileostomy. Treatment includes using a pouching system that supports both the stoma and the fistula until surgical revision can be carried out.

Parastomal Hernia

Parastomal hernia occurs with an intestinal loop protruding through a defect in the fascia around the stoma. It can result from improper siting of the stoma outside of rectus, a too-large opening into the connective tissue of the muscle, or weak abdominal muscles. Treatment includes the use of a hernia support belt. It's important to prevent constipation and evaluate stoma size while person is sitting and reclining. Colostomy irrigations should be suspended if difficulty is encountered. Surgical repair with relocation of stoma may be necessary.

Peristomal Complications

Candidiasis

Candidiasis is a common fungal infection that causes inflammation with burning, itching, and red patches, related to prolonged moisture on skin, usually from secretions or leakage under pouch. **Treatment** requires identifying and eliminating the cause of the moist environment, usually a leaking pouch. The skin should be cleaned and dried and antifungal medication applied under a properly-fitted pouch that does not allow leakage.

Folliculitis

Folliculitis is inflammation of the hair follicles by staphylococcus aureus. The lesions are often pustular, red, and painful. Folliculitis usually results from slight nicks in the skin from shaving with a razor, from friction, or from occlusion. **Treatment** includes shaving less frequently and clipping the hair or using an electric shaver. It can result from insufficient shaving, so hair is pulled out when the appliance is removed. Antibacterial soap such as chlorhexidine gluconate, may reduce infection by decreasing skin bacteria. The person should wash hands thoroughly after caring for the skin to avoid spreading the infection.

Mucosal Transplantation

Mucosal transplantation is the "transplanting" of intestinal mucosa along the suture line and onto the peristomal area, resulting from suturing through the peristomal skin rather than the stoma during the surgical procedure, leaving areas of mucosal tissue present in the peristomal area. Because these small patches of mucosa remain moist and secrete mucous, they interfere with adhesion of the pouching system. Cauterization and barrier powders will not heal the lesions because they are essentially the wrong type of tissue and cannot be changed. Excision of mucosal tissue with stoma revision is the only effective treatment.

Radiation Trauma

Radiation trauma can result in thin, friable tissue that is easily irritated and denuded by pouching systems and adhesives. Frequently the tissue is hypersensitive to chemicals in solvents or sealants, so it's best to cleanse the skin very gently with water and to avoid soaps or other irritants. Using easily removable skin barriers and pouching systems can prevent damage to skin.

Contact Dermatitis

Contact dermatitis may be either irritant or allergic. Caustic secretions may erode tissue, causing irritation, or there may be a hypersensitivity reaction to a particular chemical or product in the pouching system. Skin may be red, draining, and painful. It is necessary to determine the cause of the irritation in order to eliminate the irritant. The area of the irritation usually corresponds to the area of contact with the irritant causing the dermatitis. The pouching system may need to be changed if that is the causative agent. Reducing the use of products on the skin may help. Denuded skin may be treated with triamcinolone acetonide spray, and skin barrier powder may be used to protect the irritated skin. If the cause of the irritant is not readily discerned, then the person may need referral to a dermatologist for patch tests of various products or other skin tests of product ingredients.

Pyoderma Gangrenosum

Pyoderma gangrenosum is a condition with ulcerations that begin as pustules that form full-thickness ulcers that become inflamed and necrotic. The condition occurs in women more than men and may result from trauma or irritation from pouch adhesive. It is associated with inflammatory bowel disease, leukemia, and multiple myeloma. Treatment must address underlying disease. Topical or systemic anti-inflammatory medications may be used. Skin must be kept clean and dry with a pouching system that lasts at least 24 hours. Hydrocolloid dressings may be placed over the ulcers to use as a base for the pouch. Skin barrier powders and foam dressings may also be used for small ulcers. Wound drainage may be extensive, and this affects how long pouching system last between changes. Healing rates vary, and even after the ulcerated areas have healed, scars and uneven skin surface may make securing the pouching system difficult. Surgical resiting of the stoma may be necessary in severe cases.

Pseudoverrucous Lesions

Pseudoverrucous lesions (hyperplasia, chronic papillomatous dermatitis) are lesions resulting from chronic irritation and thickening of the epithelium caused by moisture. The number and size of lesions vary, depending upon the amount of moisture and how chronic the problem has been. The lesions are raised, wart-like, and color varies from white to red to brown. The epidermis surrounding the lesions is moist. The lesions may bleed and be painful. This condition may be caused by using a pouch with an opening that is too large. It is critical to identify and correct the cause of moisture to the skin. For urinary diversions, it helps to correct urinary pH by adequate fluid intake, cranberry juice, and Vitamin C. Lesions may be treated with vinegar soaks for 5 minutes at pouch change. Occasionally cauterization with silver nitrate on large lesions may help healing. Acidic skin barriers, such as karaya or CollySeals should be used with the pouching system.

Varices

Varices (caput medusae) are large portosystemic collateral veins that appear about the stoma, related to portal hypertension from where the portal venous system communicates with the systemic circulatory system. Varices can result from placing the stoma through the abdominal wall. Varices may result in sudden and profuse blood loss, with blood usually noted in the pouch or around the stoma when the pouch is changed. Development of varices is most common in people with liver malignancies and those with an inflammatory bowel disease treated with ileostomy and proctocolectomy. Direct pressure is used to stop bleeding, followed by cauterization, or suturing. A piece-pouching system is used to avoid pressure during application. Surgical treatment may be needed, including ligation of the portosystemic channels, creation of a portosystemic shunt to lower pressure, or liver transplantation. Person should be educated about signs of bleeding and first aid measures to stop bleeding until emergency help arrives.

Suture Granulomas

Suture granulomas are granulation tissue at the skin-stoma base as a reaction to retained or reactive sutures. They appear as erythematous, friable lesions that bleed easily. They are usually small and round and scattered about the suture line. Remove sutures. It's important to identify any retained sutures and remove them. Silver nitrate cauterization may be needed to decrease the amount of tissue. Surgical cauterization may be necessary in severe cases.

Trauma

Trauma is skin injury with loss of epidermis. It usually affects small areas, but people who are sensitive to adhesive may develop sensitivity that results in sloughing of surface skin. It is often related to irritation caused by removal of tape from the skin, but it may also be caused by an insecure appliance and pressure of belt or clothes as well as incorrect shaving. It is necessary to determine the cause of the trauma and eliminate it. Skin barriers may be needed to protect skin during healing.

Atypical Stoma and Peristomal Complications

Some atypical stomal/peristomal complications include:

- **Malignancy** at stoma site can happen as a result of implantation during surgical procedure or incomplete resection of tumor. Peristomal cancer is rare and may result from chronic skin irritation. Surgical revision with wide excision and re-siting of the stoma is treatment of choice.
- **Herpes zoster and herpes simplex**, viral illnesses, remain dormant but can be triggered by illness or stress. Antiviral treatments may be used. Herpetic lesions in the peristomal area may be irritated by pouch adhesive. Hydrocolloid dressing may be used to prevent fluid from lesions from interfering with the pouching system.
- **Pemphigus** is an autoimmune skin disease causing blistering and affecting peristomal skin, requiring referral to dermatologist, who may treat with corticosteroids, dapsone, or mycophenolate mofetil. It may require temporary use of non-adhesive pouch with hydrocolloid or foam dressings as base.
- **Psoriasis** is a condition with painful crusted scaly plaques, requiring referral to dermatologist for medications to control lesions that interfere with pouch adhesion.

Possible Postoperative Complications with Fecal and Urinary Diversion Procedures

Postoperative complications from a fecal/urinary diversion placement include the following:

- **Ileus** is paralysis of the bowel causing absence of bowel sounds and inability to pass flatus or stool, associated with abdominal discomfort and distention.
- **Anastomotic leak** is leakage from surgical site associated with distention and signs of infection. Leakage is most common in unstable or malnourished patients or those with fecal contamination of wound. It may be related to poor siting of stoma in a location close to bones, near old scars, or along the main incision, resulting in irritation.
- **Hemorrhage** may indicate the mesenteric vessel is open, requiring surgical intervention to repair damage.
- **Ischemia** is characterized by cyanotic discoloration of the stoma and may range from sloughing of mucosa to necrosis of tissue. It results from interruption of blood flow from numerous causes, such as too much tension on the mesentery, excessive mesentery stripping, or constrictive sutures.
- **Mucocutaneous separation** is an opening between the stoma and the skin where the sutures have separated.

Reanastomosis/Takedown of Colostomy

For a reanastomosis/takedown of a colostomy, an incision is made around the stoma to separate it from the abdominal wall. Next, the proximal bowel segment is reattached to the distal segment. Finally, the abdominal wound is closed.

Complications include:

- **Anastomotic leak**: Occasionally there is a leak at the site of the anastomosis, causing fecal material to leak into the abdominal cavity and posing a danger of peritonitis.
- **Fascia dehiscence**: The fibrous tissue may split apart.
- **Wound infection**: Infection of the wound at the site of the reattachment or at the skin level can occur, especially in people who are compromised because of age or health.
- **Pulmonary complications**: Pneumonia and/or atelectasis may develop as a result of any surgery, so patients should be encouraged to stop smoking prior to surgery and to do deep-breathing/cough exercises.
- **Ileus/small bowel obstruction**: Any manipulation of the bowel may result in paralysis or obstruction of the bowel.
- **Hernia**: Post-surgical hernia may occur at surgical site.

Fistulae

Fistula and Terminology Related to Fistulas

A fistula is an abnormal passage or tunnel from one internal organ to another or from an internal organ to the body surface. There may be multiple branches from a fistula rather than just one tunnel. Fistulas may be blind (only one open end), complete (openings both internally and externally), or incomplete (external skin opening with no connection to an internal organ).

- **Anorectal**: From the rectum or other anorectal area to the skin.
- **Colocutaneous**: From the colon to the skin surface.
- **Colovesical**: From the colon to the bladder.
- **Enterocolonic**: From the small intestine to the colon.
- **Enterocutaneous**: From the small intestine to the skin surface.
- **Enteroenteral**: Between two parts of the intestine.
- **Enterovaginal**: From the small intestine to the vagina.
- **Enterovesical**: From the small intestine to the bladder.
- **Rectovaginal**: From the rectum to the vagina.
- **Vesicocutaneous**: From the bladder to the skin surface.
- **Vesicovaginal**: From the bladder to the vagina.

Classification Systems for Fistulas

Classification systems for fistulas help to characterize the fistula and assist in the management and treatment. Sometimes, more than one classification may be used. For example, a fistula may be described as "Complex, Type I with small to medium output."

Simple/Complex

Simple fistulas are short and direct tracts with no organ involvement or abscess. **Complex, Type I fistulas** involve multiple organs with an abscess associated. **Complex, Type II fistulas** open into the base of a disrupted wound.

Volume

With this classification system, the fistula is classified according to the amount of drainage from the wound in a 24-hour period. Low-output fistulas drain less than 150 mL per 24 hours. Small to medium output fistulas drain 150-500 mL per 24 hours, and high output fistulas drain more than 500 mL per 24 hours.

Pseudostoma

A pseudostoma is an unintended, nonsurgical opening on the abdominal wall that resembles a stoma. The pseudostoma most often results from a chronic enterocutaneous fistula although it can also occur at a prior stoma site. Patients with Crohn disease are especially at risk. Once a fistula forms, the channel is narrow and lined with granulation tissue, which begins to epithelialize. The drainage causes chemical irritation and maceration of surrounding tissue at the drainage site. In time, the segment of the bowel that is attached to the fistula adheres to the inner abdominal wall and the tract widens. The bowel may prolapse into the tract and through the fistula opening, where is mimics the appearance of a stoma. The tissue about the pseudostoma often becomes very inflamed and macerated, and drainage is often irregular. Management of the pseudostoma is similar to that of other fistulae: application of wound management system, peristomal skin protection, nutrition, hydration, and emotional support. A pseudostoma rarely heals spontaneously but requires surgical intervention when inflammation recedes. Preventive measures include reducing fistula output, closure of the fistula and/or wound surrounding the fistula. and protecting the skin from drainage.

Acute/Chronic Fistulae

The differences between acute and chronic fistulae are shown below:

Acute	Chronic
• Newly-formed, less than 4–6 weeks. • Surrounding tissue inflamed, friable, necrotic. • Tract immature. • Pain intense and acute. • Etiology: surgery, trauma, infection. • High potential for spontaneous closure if underlying cause corrected. • Increased risk of abscess, sepsis, electrolyte imbalance.	• Longstanding with failure to close, more than 4–6 weeks. • Surrounding tissue fibrotic, epithelialized, scarred. • Tract mature, epithelialization present. • Pain chronic. • Etiology: Unresolved acute fistula, Crohn's disease • Low potential for spontaneous closure. • Increased risk of skin maceration, malnutrition, chronic inflammation.

Fistulae most at risk for chronicity include enterocutaneous, enterovesical, rectovaginal, and cholecystoduodenal although any type of fistula can become chronic. Fistulae are likely to become chronic if any FRIEND factors are present: **F** (foreign body), **R** (radiation-damaged tissue, **I** (infection/inflammation), **E** (epithelialization), **N** (neoplasm), and **D** (distal obstruction).

Parks Classification System for Anorectal Fistulas

Parks classification system for anorectal fistulas classifies four different types of cryptoglandular (pertaining to the anal glands) fistulas. Anorectal fistulas are the most common type of fistula, occurring most frequently in women.

- **Intersphincteric fistulas** extend from the internal sphincter downward to the perineum, up to a high blind tract, or open into the rectum itself (70%).
- **Transsphincteric fistulas** extend from the internal and external sphincters to the ischiorectal fossa to the perineum (25%).
- **Suprasphincteric fistulas** cross the internal sphincter to the external sphincter above the puborectalis muscles and then down to the ischioanal fossa and to the skin (5%).
- **Extrasphincteric fistulas** extend from the perianal skin through the levator ani muscles and through the rectal wall (1%).

An additional classification is sometimes added to the original four:

- **Horseshoe fistulas** partially circle the anus, opening at both ends in the cutaneous tissue.

Assessing Drainage from Fistulas

Considerations when assessing the drainage from fistulas include:

- **Source of fistula**, whether it is near wound, stoma, organ, or bony prominence, helps determine the type of discharge. Enzymatic drainage, as from enterocutaneous fistula, may be corrosive to the tissue.
- **Type of drainage** includes color, consistency, and odor. Color of purulent discharge is often yellow, light brown, or slightly green. Fecal material draining through a fistula may range in color from golden (from the jejunum) or brown (from the descending colon), depending on fistula location.
- **Consistency** may range from very watery to very thick. Urinary discharge through a fistula may be combined with purulent material and mucous, and may be thin in consistency. Odor from fecal material, especially from the lower colon, is noticeable. Some types of infection have a pronounced foul odor. Odor in discharge is always a cause for concern.
- **Amount of drainage** is important for choosing the type of dressings and need for electrolyte replacement.

Percutaneous Tubes

Nasogastric Tubes, Sump Tubes, and Levin Tubes

Nasogastric tubes (NG) are plastic or vinyl tubes inserted through the nose, down esophagus, and into the stomach.

Sump tubes are radiopaque with a vent lumen to prevent a vacuum from forming with high suction.

Levin tubes have no vent lumen and are used only with low suction.

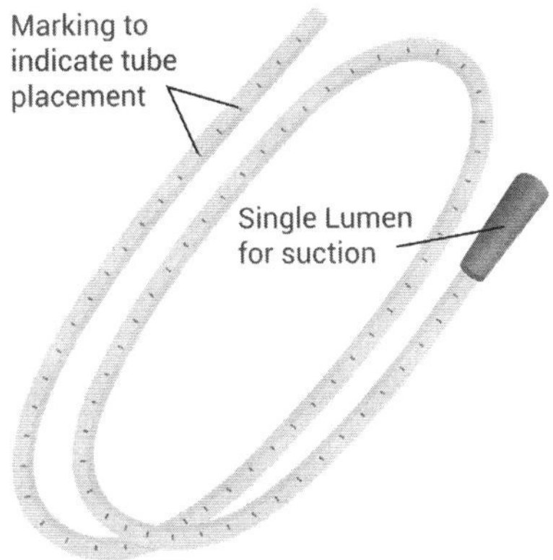

Levin Tube

The purpose of nasogastric tubes is to drain gastric secretions, allow sampling of secretions, or provide access to the stomach and upper gastrointestinal tract. They are used for lavage after medication overdose, for decompression, for instillation of medications or fluids. Nasogastric tubes should not be used if there is obstruction proximal to the stomach or gastric pathology, such as hemorrhage.

Management involves securing the tube at a downward angle, avoiding pressure on the nares that could lead to irritation or ulceration, providing drainage tubing and bags for gravity drainage if indicated, and monitoring drainage. Tubes attached to continuous low or intermittent high suction must be monitored frequently.

Extended Use Nasogastric Tubes and Intestinal Tubes

Extended use nasogastric tubes or small-bore feeding tubes are flexible with weighted tips to maintain placement. These are often inserted with help of a guidewire. The purpose is to provide gastric access for temporary tube feedings. **Management** includes checking patency and flushing on a regular schedule because small lumen is easily occluded. The tube must be taped securely and angled downward, avoiding pressure on the nares that could lead to ulceration.

Intestinal tubes are longer tubes, reaching beyond the duodenum, up to 10 feet and weighted at the end with a mercury- or tungsten-filled balloon so the tube will advance through the intestine. The Cantor tube is a 10-foot single lumen tube. The Miller-Abbot tube is a double-lumen tube with an inflatable balloon that is inflated after tube is in the stomach. The purpose is decompression for bowel obstruction. **Management** includes instructing patient on positions to advance tube, securing tube, and monitoring drainage.

Nephrostomy Tubes

Nephrostomy tubes are inserted into the kidney pelvis to provide drainage. The nephrostomy tube is inserted in the flank area, near the kidney, and drains through extension tubing into a bedside urinary bag or leg bag. The purpose of the tube is to provide drainage for urine and prevent hydronephrosis when there is a blockage in the urinary system. It may be used for kidney stones, cancer, strictures, stent placement, or to allow healing of a distal portion of the urinary tract. The tube may be inserted temporarily or permanently. **Management** includes irrigating with 5-10 mL of sterile water if necessary, securing the tube with sutures or attachment devices, keeping the surrounding skin dry and clean, observing for signs of complications (fever, chills, flank pain, tube leakage, blood or purulent drainage or discharge), and educating patient about the care of the tube and use and care of drainage tubes and bags.

Biliary Tubes

Biliary tubes or t-tubes are placed surgically in the liver and bile ducts to promote biliary drainage. The purpose of biliary tubes is to provide drainage, prevent blockage, serve as a stent for perforations, and allow easy access to laboratory sampling of discharge. They are used before or after surgical procedures such as liver transplants or complicated cholecystectomy. Either biliary tubes or stents may be used for decompression after common bile duct exploration. **Management** includes securing tube, measuring output, preventing backflow by maintaining gravity drainage system, keeping skin clean with normal saline and drying to prevent irritation, irrigating the drains as necessary to prevent blockage, observing for signs of infection (fever, chills, bile leakage around tube, bloody or purulent drainage or discharge), and educating the patient about the caring for the tube. Drainage after liver transplant should be observed carefully for inspissated (thickened) biliary sludge, indicating necrosis of bile duct walls.

Drains

Simple drains are latex or vinyl tubes of varying sizes and lengths inserted into a wound to provide drainage of serous material, blood, pus, or other discharge. This type of drain is usually placed through a stab wound near the area of involvement or at a surgical site. An example is a **Jackson Pratt drain**, which uses a bulb that is attached to the drainage tube to create suction. The bulb collects fluid and must be emptied when full. The suction is created by squeezing the bulb with the stopper open, then closing the stopper so there is negative pressure in the bulb and tubing.

JACKSON PRATT DRAIN

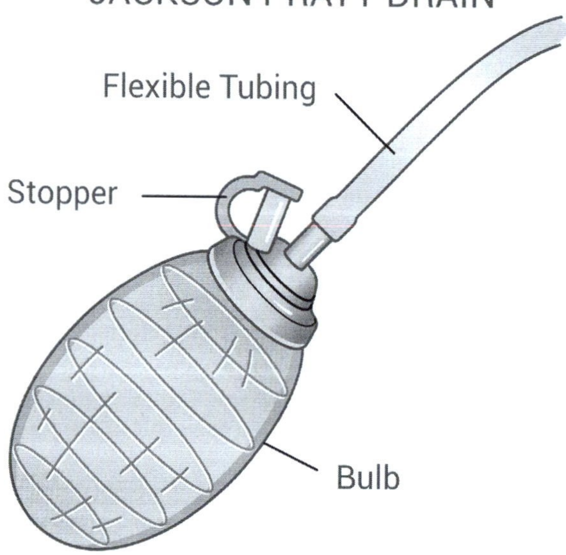

Penrose drains are soft rubber/latex tubes that are flat in appearance and are placed in surgical wounds to drain fluid by gravity and capillary action. They are available in various diameters and lengths.

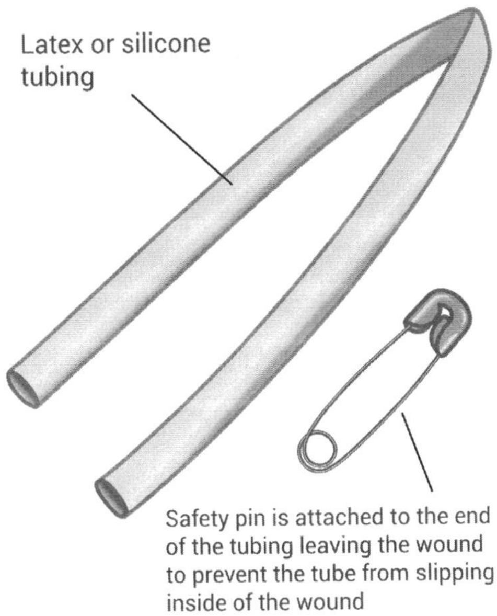

Penrose Drain

Sump drains are double-lumen or tri-lumen tubes (with a third lumen for infusions). A large outflow lumen and small inflow lumen produces venting when air enters the inflow lumen and forces drainage into the large lumen.

Percutaneous drainage catheter is inserted into wound to provide continuous drainage for infection or symptoms from collection of drainage in the wound. Irrigation of the catheter may need to be done to maintain patency. Skin barriers and pouching systems may be necessary.

SAFE PERCUTANEOUS DRAINAGE KIT

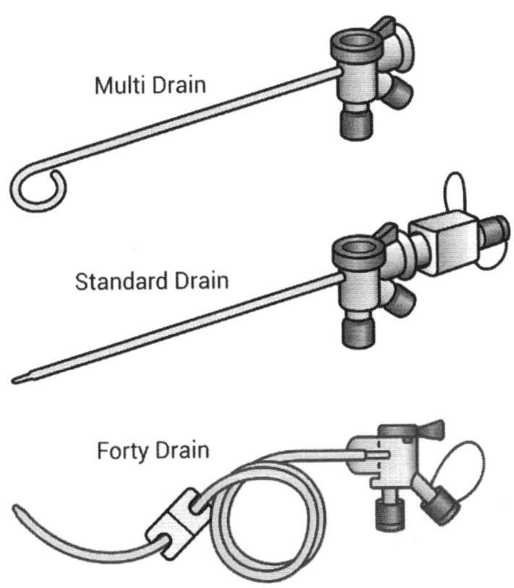

Important Terms

Agenesis: The failure of an organ to grow or develop properly.

Atresia: Congenital absence or closure of an orifice or tubular structure.

Exstrophy: A congenital eversion (turning inside out) of an organ.

Extrusion: Protruding externally in an abnormal manner.

Fistula: An abnormal passage, tube-like structure, or opening between 2 internal structures or between an internal structure and the body surface.

Gangrene/dry gangrene: Loss of blood supply resulting in death of tissue, often allowing bacterial invasion. Dry gangrene does not involve bacterial infection of tissue, only necrosis.

Inspissation/inspissated: Condition of thickening/thick.

Ischemia: Lack of adequate blood supply to a local area due to obstruction of blood vessels, resulting in inadequate oxygen and nutrient supply to the tissue.

Necrosis: Death of cells or tissue because of insufficient blood flow, injury, disease, or other pathology.

Perforation: The condition of a hole through the wall of an organ or body structure.

Intervention and Treatment

Colostomy Management

One- or Two-Piece Pouching Systems

The procedures for one- and two-piece pouch systems are as follows:

1. Assemble supplies/equipment.
2. Empty pouch into toilet.
3. Gently remove pouch, working from the top down, using one hand to pull the pouch away from the skin and the other to push down on skin. Save clamp and place used pouch in a plastic bag.
4. Cleanse skin with water and examine for irritation or lesions. Dry. Shave if necessary with electric shaver.
5. Examine stoma and measure if necessary.
6. Cut appliance to fit if necessary or use precut appliance if stoma is round. Remove paper backing from appliance. Apply starting from the bottom, fitting under the stoma first and then smoothing upward so the warmth of the hands helps the appliance to adhere. If two-piece appliance, apply pouch to skin barrier.
7. Apply tape at corners of pouch if necessary.
8. Place ostomy deodorant in fecal pouch if desired and then apply clamp/close spout.

Stoma Site Location

The site of the stoma is influence by the purpose. For example, a permanent colostomy will likely be in the left ileac fossa while an ileostomy stoma will likely be in the right iliac fossa. The placement of the stoma should take into consideration what will be most convenient for the patient, collect drainage effectively, and not leak or damage the skin. There should be adequate space about the stoma for adherence of an appliance, allowing for at least 2.5 inches of flat adhesive surface for pouching. Areas that should be avoided include about the waistline and groin areas because bending would loosen the appliance and cause discomfort. Appliances will not adhere properly to skin folds, scars, bony prominences, and about the umbilicus because the surfaces are not adequately flat. When siting the stoma, the patient should be both in standing and sitting position because the abdominal contours may change. The patient should be able to see and reach the appliance easily. Additionally, the patient should wear and appliance over the chosen site for at least 24 hours to determine if it is satisfactory. Patients may need guidance in the type of clothing that helps to camouflage appliances and that allow for easy access, including loose shirts and dresses.

Marking the Stoma Site

The three methods for marking the stoma site are explained below:

- **Permanent marker**: Site is marked with an X or circle, and usually covered with a transparent dressing to protect the markings. Markings will usually last for 1-3 weeks, but patients should be provided a marking pen and additional dressings in case markings fade.
- **Tattoo**: Target site is cleansed with alcohol, India ink is dropped on the site, and the skin is punctured 3 times with a small-gauge needle. The area is then cleansed and dressed. An alternate tattooing procedure is to inject a small amount of methylene blue (0.01 mL) intradermally. Tattooing is the most permanent method but is painful for the patient.

- **Laceration**: Site is marked by making circular scratches in the epidermis with a small-gauge needle. This method is not recommended because the break in the skin can lead to infection. However, some surgeons use this method prior to the surgical scrub to ensure that markings remain through scrub.

Modifications in Procedure for Marking the Stoma Site

Modifications in procedure for marking the stoma site in special circumstances are discussed below:

- **Thinness/cachexia**: If recent weight loss, person may regain weight, affecting stoma siting. Skin turgor may be poor.
- **Obesity/abdominal distension**: Follow nipple line down to abdomen to site stoma if rectus muscle non-palpable. If necessary, place stoma in upper quadrant to allow patient access. Evaluate females with large breasts in sitting position with and without bras to see if breasts obscure stoma site.
- **Physical considerations**:
    - Wheelchair bound should be evaluated in wheelchair.
    - Kyphosis or lordosis affects placement and people may benefit from wearing pouch for 24 hours to assure adherence.
    - Sports enthusiasts/physical laborers should be asked to go through the motions of their activities to make sure stoma is sited to avoid irritation.
- **Pediatric concerns**: avoiding umbilical cord area in newborns. Parents should be with children, and nurse should use an ostomy-teaching doll.
- **Post-radiation**: Post-radiation tissue may be damaged, so radiated area should be avoided.
- **Fecal and urinary diversions**: Both fecal and urinary diversions require that stomas be sited on different planes in case one pouch needs to be belted.

Minimizing Odor from Stoma and Pouch

Proper pouching is important because improper pouching is the cause of most odors:

- **Fecal diversions**: Check pouch for leaks. Check closure to verify it is clean and no fecal material has leaked around the opening. Make sure clamp is clean and secure. Avoid putting holes in appliance for release of gas as leaking gas may have a foul odor. Empty pouch regularly, using proper procedures.
- **Urinary diversions**: Wipe off end of spout to remove drops of remaining urine. Replace connecting tubing and bedside or leg bags, usually not odor proof, if odor develops.

Diet control includes avoiding gas/odor-producing foods.

- Fecal diversions:
    - **Vegetables**: cabbage, broccoli, kale, cauliflower, kohlrabi, Brussels sprouts, asparagus, onions, dried peas, rutabagas, turnips. Proteins: dried beans fish, strong cheeses, and eggs.
    - **Other**: spicy foods, chewing gum. Drinks: beer, carbonated beverages (such as sodas or juices).
- Urinary diversions:
    - Asparagus, fish, various spices.

Colostomy Irrigation

The procedures for colostomy irrigation are as follows:

1. Gather all equipment, fill irrigating bag with lukewarm water (500-1500 mL), release air bubbles from tubing, and hang with bottom of bag at shoulder level.
2. Sit on or next to toilet and apply long irrigation sleeve, placing the end into the toilet.
3. Lubricate cone nozzle and insert into stoma (usually about 3 inches) in direction of colon.
4. Holding cone firmly in place to retain fluid, open clamp and let fluid flow into colon slowly over about 5-10 minutes. Hold cone in place for a few seconds, and then remove.
5. Drain fecal output into toilet for 10-15 minutes. Initial flow of fluids is usually followed by fecal material within 15 minutes.
6. Dry end of irrigation sleeve and clamp. Keep bag in place for up to an hour if stool continues to drain. Remove irrigation sleeve, cleanse peristomal area, and apply pouch.
7. Cleanse irrigation equipment.

Management of Retained Distal Segment of Bowel for Colostomy Patients

Management of retained distal segments depends to some degree on whether or not further surgery is planned to reattach the colon. General observations for signs of infection are especially important: fever, distention, and change in bowel habits.

- **Loop colostomy**: Loop of bowel brought to abdominal surface but not completely severed, usually with a rod holding loop above skin. Intestinal loop is cut partially open, creating two stomas—a proximal for fecal drainage and a small distal mucous fistula. Cleanse mucous fistula of discharge.
- **End-loop (double-barrel) colostomy with mucous fistula**: Portion of colon removed; both proximal and distal ends are brought through abdominal wall, creating two stomas, proximal for stool and distal for mucus.
- **Management**: Mucous fistulas should be cleansed with gauze and discharge examined for blood and/or pus or any other changes in character. Cleanse peristomal area carefully to prevent irritation. If rectum in place, check rectal area for irritation and discharge.

Relationship Between Placement of Colostomy and Character of Stool

Ascending colon: Because the stool is in liquid or semi-liquid form coming from the small intestine, it is still quite liquid or pasty in nature in the ascending colon. Diarrhea is the primary complication.

Transverse colon: With some of the fluid absorbed, the stool in the transverse colon is semi-liquid to soft, depending in part on the placement, right or left, of the stoma and the amount of transverse colon remaining. Diarrhea is the more common complication although constipation can occur, especially if much of the transverse colon is intact.

Descending colon: Much of the fluid has been reabsorbed from the stool by the time it reaches the descending colon, so the stool is semi-formed and soft. Diarrhea can occur as well as constipation.

Sigmoid colon: Reabsorption of fluids in the colon has been completed and the stool is fully formed. Diarrhea can occur, but constipation is a more common problem.

LAXATIVE AND ANTIFLATULENT AGENTS FOR THOSE WITH FECAL DIVERSION

The following are laxative and antiflatulent agents that may be helpful to those with fecal diversion:

- **Laxative agents**: Osmotic (Milk of Magnesia) and stimulant (Dulcolax) laxatives should not be taken by those with ileostomies as they can lead to increased diarrhea and electrolyte imbalance. They should be rarely used by others and only with the advice of healthcare providers. Overuse can lead to bowel dysfunction.
- **Fiber/bulk agents**: These agents dissolve or swell in the intestines, promoting peristalsis and include preparations made with methylcellulose (Citrucel), psyllium (Metamucil), and bran. These can reduce diarrhea and help with constipation.
- **Stool softeners**: These increase retention of fluid in the stool (DSS, Colace), helping to prevent constipation and impaction.
- **Antiflatulent agents**: These agents both disperse gas and prevent formation of gas bubbles. Simethicone (Phazyme) allows small gas bubbles to gather into larger ones, making them easier to expel by belching. The food enzyme alpha-galactosidase (Beano), which prevents gas related only to complex sugars but not sorbitol, lactose, fiber, or wheat.

Ileostomy Management

Management of Retained Distal Segment of Bowel with Ileostomies

Management of retained distal segments varies according to procedures completed or planned. In the case of complete proctocolectomy, the focus will simply be on healing because the distal segments have been excised. If reattachment or creation of a reservoir is planned, then distal segments must be monitored.

- **Loop ileostomy**: Loop of ileum brought to abdominal surface but not completely severed, usually with a rod holding loop above skin. Intestinal loop is cut partially open, creating two stomas—a proximal for fecal drainage and a small distal mucous fistula. Cleanse mucous discharge and check mucous fistula when pouch changed.
- **Ileostomy with ileoanal, J, S, or W pouch**: Monitor any discharge, distention, pain, fever, or other signs of infection. If anus intact, observe drainage for signs of infection. Cleanse perianal area and provide protective cream or ointment to prevent irritation. If pouch is created before closure of ileostomy, observe for pouchitis.

Continent Ileostomy

Drainage and Management of Kock Pouch

A **Kock pouch** uses the lower part of the small bowel to create an internal reservoir (pouch) for the collection of fecal material. This pouch is created from the small intestine and has a leak-free nipple valve inside the abdominal stoma, created by intussuscepting a portion of the ileal loop back through the ileum, to prevent leakage of stool, with an intestinal conduit leading to the pouch.

- **Draining**: Insert plastic catheter about 5 inches into stoma and lower opposite end of catheter over toilet to drain. Initially, pouch must be drained about every 3 hours because capacity is small. After about 2 months, pouch needs to be drained only 3-5 times a day.
- **Management**: Avoid eating late in the evening so pouch won't need draining during the night. Diet modification can prevent constipation or diarrhea. The stoma, about 1/2 inch in diameter, is covered with gauze or stoma cap to absorb mucus. Irrigate as directed, usually twice daily.

Draining

General procedures for draining the continent ileostomy in the initial postoperative phase and in later weeks and months are explained below:

- **Initial 3-4 weeks**: Prevent excessive pressure that could cause perforation or tearing by using constant drainage. If catheter plugs or falls out, replace immediately. The catheter needs to be irrigated with 1 ounce of tap water several times daily, letting liquid drain back out.
- **Next phase**: Continuous draining stops and intermittent draining begins, usually every 2 hours during the day with constant drainage at night. Pouch should be drained first thing in the morning and last thing at night. Gradually the time interval between draining increases and constant night drainage stops, but the pouch may need to be drained once or twice during the night.
- **3 months later**: The pouch should be well healed and functioning. Usual practice is to drain the pouch 4-6 times a day and irrigate 2 of these times. Any time there is a feeling of being full, bloated, or distended, the pouch should be drained as well as before physical activity.

Irrigating

The procedure for irrigating continent ileostomy is described below:

1. Gather supplies.
2. Remove dressing/stoma cap and discard.
3. Insert catheter if not in place.
4. Fill syringe with 30 mL of tap water, insert it into end of catheter, and inject with gentle pressure only.
5. Pinch the catheter to prevent drainage, remove the syringe, and then unpinch the catheter and allow it to drain into a basin or the toilet bowl.
6. The irrigation may need to be repeated until the stool flows back freely.
7. DO NOT use the syringe to pull the stool or fluid back out. Always allow it to drain back out by gravity.
8. If liquid drains back very slowly, the catheter may be blocked; remove, rinse with tap water, and reinsert.
9. DO NOT put more than 60 mL of water into pouch without ensuring the fluid is draining out.
10. Remove catheter, cleanse skin, and reapply stoma dressing.

Prevention for Fluid and Electrolyte Imbalance with an Ileostomy

Causes of fluid/electrolyte imbalance: After the large intestine is removed, the body adjusts by absorbing more fluids and nutrients in the small intestine, and the stool becomes thicker, increasing the danger of dehydration. Bouts of diarrhea with excessively watery stools can also lead to dehydration and electrolyte imbalance. With electrolyte imbalance, just increasing the oral intake of fluids is not sufficient as these fluids will be excreted through the kidneys and may not correct the electrolyte imbalance. Excessive heat can also cause dehydration and electrolyte imbalance. All types of fluid loss involve loss of electrolytes.

Signs and symptoms include:

- Mouth/tongue dry. Skin turgor poor.
- Weight loss. Diarrhea. Lethargy.

Strategies for prevention are as follows:

- Maintain adequate fluid and nutritional intake.
- Estimate/monitor intake and output.
- Monitor weight.
- Drink Gatorade or other such liquids with diarrhea or dehydration.
- If stool too liquid, increase fibrous foods; too dry, increase salty foods.
- Antidiarrheal agents may be necessary.
- Lavage.

Mechanical Obstruction of an Ileostomy

Causes of mechanical obstruction: Obstruction of an ileostomy is almost always food-related. After the large intestine is removed, the body adjusts by absorbing more fluids and nutrients in the small intestine; the stool becomes thicker, increasing the danger of dehydration. Mechanical obstruction is almost always caused by high fiber foods, such as inadequately-chewed popcorn, nuts, celery, coconut, and corn. This mass causes the bowel above to become hyperactive as it contracts, trying to move the mass of fiber. As the pressure builds, the part of the intestine below the mass may collapse, causing a reverse peristalsis.

Signs and symptoms include:

- Edematous stoma. High-pitched bowel sounds.
- Obvious peristaltic waves. Nausea and vomiting.
- Abdominal pain. Distention.
- Dry mouth, loss of skin turgor. Watery diarrhea.

Strategies of prevention are as follows:

- Increase fluids and avoid dehydration.
- High fiber foods should be taken in limited quantities and chewed thoroughly.
- Warm bath may relax abdominal muscles.
- Drink warm fluids and assume the knee-chest position.

Lavage of an Ileostomy to Relieve Blockage

Lavage is usually done after an abdominal x-ray has determined that food is the cause of the blockage. It is NOT the same as an irrigation, which uses large volumes of fluid. Normal saline (NS) is used to prevent further dehydration, instilled with a catheter-tipped piston or bulb syringe with a 14-16 Fr catheter attached. The procedure is done to "flush" the blockage loose.

1. Gather supplies.
2. Remove pouching system and apply irrigation sleeve with end in toilet (or bedpan).
3. Do a digital exam to determine direction of intestine.
4. Lubricate the catheter and gently insert approximately 12-15 cms.
5. Slowly inject 30-50 mL of normal saline into the intestine and then slowly aspirate the entire amount with light to moderate pressure.
6. Repeat the procedure of flushing with normal saline until the blockage is relieved.
7. Measure the stoma (because of swelling) and apply the correctly-sized pouch.

Ileostomy Takedown

Usually about two months after the temporary ileostomy, the ileostomy is closed and the proximal and distal segments are reattached/opened for intestinal continuity. The ileoanal reservoir is usually quite small after surgery, so 8-10 stools per day is not unusual, but the reservoir capacity will expand and stool frequency will decrease over a 6- to 12-month period. The best functional results would be 4-5 stools per day with no incontinence. Most current procedures result in 95% continence during the day and 90% during the night.

Complications are as follows:

- **Wound infection**: May be superficial at abdominal surface or at anastomosis.
- **Small bowel obstruction**: Usually corrected non-surgically.
- **Anastomotic leak**: Can lead to serious infection/peritonitis.
- **GI bleeding from peri-anastomotic ulcers**: Sometimes arises from side to side anastomosis of small bowel for pouch formation.
- **Steroids**: Can increase wound complications, so wean steroids prior to surgery.
- **Pouchitis**: Non-specific inflammation of pouch, usually in the first two years.

Urostomy Management

Ureteral Stent and Post-Surgical Management

Ureteral stent: A piece of thin pliable tubing that is inserted inside of the ureter to maintain patency, during post-surgical period when edema of the ureter could cause occlusion. These tubes protrude through the stoma and are often different lengths or color-coded to differentiate which ureter they serve.

Post-surgical management: Ureteral stents are usually removed after 5 to 7 days although they may be left in for several weeks. Each protruding stent should be drained separately and clearly labeled. Stents have multiple holes along the length of the tube to promote drainage. Ensure that the stents are not dislodged or blocked. If pain, purulent discharge, or fever occurs, a chest x-ray may be taken to determine position of the stent. Patient must be advised NOT to remove the stent. The stent may be irrigated with 5-10 mL of normal saline, using care not to apply tension or pressure that may dislodge the tube.

Changing and Managing Urostomy Pouch

The two main types of **urostomy pouches** are the one-piece with attached skin barrier and the two-piece with a skin barrier and pouch that detaches. The pouches have drains at the bottom for emptying and to attach a nighttime drainage tube.

- **Changing the pouch**: If possible, change pouch in the morning before eating or drinking when urine flow is decreased, or wait 2 hours after eating or drinking. Remove pouch. Stand or sit as comfortable, keeping a paper towel or gauze to absorb drops of urine. Cleanse peristomal tissue, dry skin, and apply new bag, using a mirror to guide if necessary.
- **Emptying the pouch**: Empty the pouch regularly to prevent bacteria from growing in the urine, usually every 2-4 hours during the day. Children may need more frequent draining because the pouch is smaller. Empty the pouch when it is about 1/3 full. Open the valve at the bottom and drain directly into a toilet or other container.

Modifications and Management for Urostomies

Fluid modifications: Adequate intake of fluids is critical to prevent urinary complications, such as infections. Oral intake should be 2000-2500 mL (8-10 glasses) per day.

Nighttime management: To prevent the ostomy bag from becoming overfull during the night and pulling away from the skin, a long tube should attach a large overnight urinary drainage bag. The bag can be placed in a container on the floor or hung on the side of the bed. Overnight drainage also helps to keep the urine from constantly bathing the stoma and causing white, gritty crystals to form. Acidifying the urine by taking vitamin C can treat these crystals.

Mucus management: Mucus in urine is usually managed by increasing fluids to flush the mucus. In immediate post-surgical period, a marked increase in mucus in the urine may occur but will usually abate. Gentle irrigations will be done post-surgically to maintain patency of catheters.

Protecting the Peristomal Tissue with a Urostomy

Pouching: Measure the stoma and make sure that the opening in the skin barrier is the correct size. Drain on a regular schedule to avoid leaks, and change the pouch regularly before leaks occur.

Protect skin: Remove the pouch and cleanse the skin immediately if there is pain, itching, or burning in peristomal area. Use care when removing the skin barrier so that the skin does not pull. Put pressure on the skin to push it away from the barrier. Wash peristomal skin carefully with water and mild soap if necessary or shower after the pouch is removed. Be sure that peristomal skin is thoroughly dry before applying barrier.

Observe: Check area carefully and be aware that sensitivities and allergies to adhesives, barriers, or material in pouches can develop over time. It may be necessary to try different types of barriers or to use a pouch cover to protect the skin.

Continent Diversion

Irrigating the Urinary Reservoir for Continent Cutaneous Urinary Diversions

Irrigation of the urinary reservoir is done frequently in the immediate post-operative period. The person with the urinary reservoir (or a care giver) should be taught irrigate in preparation for leaving the hospital.

1. Gather supplies, wash hands.
2. Remove dressing or stoma cap if one is in place.
3. Insert catheter into reservoir (unless a catheter is still in place for continuous drainage), NEVER force; drain urine.
4. Attach syringe to end of catheter and gently aspirate to make sure the reservoir is empty.
5. Draw 60 mL of sterile water/normal saline into syringe, insert syringe into catheter end, and gently inject the fluid.
6. Keep catheter elevated or pinched to prevent drainage and inject another 40 mL of water to a total of 100 mL.
7. Gently aspirate to begin flow and then allow fluid to drain by gravity.
8. Repeat irrigation if necessary until urine is clear if there is excessive mucus.

Management of Mucus for Continent Cutaneous Urinary Diversions

In the immediate post-operative period, the urinary reservoir and the intestinal conduit produce large amounts of mucus, giving the urine a cloudy appearance and creating sediment or long strands of mucoid-appearing material. Mucus is usually white and can be differentiated from yellow or greenish purulent material that indicates an infection. However, any cloudiness in urine should be suspect and requires careful observation. While a catheter is in place after surgery, it may be gently irrigated maintain patency and to prevent blockage, which could put stress on the reservoir and damage the suture lines. After the catheter is removed, increasing fluid intake to 8 to 10 glasses a day can reduce the amount of mucus. Additionally, people will need to irrigate the reservoir every 4-6 hours with small amounts of sterile water for the first 3 weeks and later as directed by their physician to empty reservoir of large amounts of mucus.

Selection of Appropriate Intubation and Dressing Supplies

Catheters: The size of the catheter used will depend to some degree on the type of nipple valve. Most people will need a 16-18 Fr straight catheter, but some tighter valves may need a 10-14 Fr catheter. Most catheters are 16 inches long, allowing for drainage into the toilet while the person is sitting on the toilet. Some catheters are latex free, some plastic, and some rubber. A clear catheter makes observation of the draining urine easier than an opaque catheter.

Irrigating syringe: A 60-70 mL injection or bulb syringe is necessary for irrigation.

Sterile water/normal saline: These solutions may be purchased or may be prepared at home.

Dressing supplies: There is a wide range of choices, including absorbent pads with hypoallergenic adhesives, and stoma caps in various shapes and sizes (look like flesh-colored adhesive bandages). Nursing pads/eye pads are inexpensive, easily available substitutions for stoma dressings.

Incontinence After Catheter Removal for Those with an Orthotopic Neobladder

Urinate on a regularly scheduled basis with straining as the bladder may not have the normal sensation of fullness:

- **First week**: Every 2 hours during the day and 3 hours during the night.
- **Second week**: Every 3 hours during the day and 4 hours during the night.
- **Third week and later**: Every 4 hours during the day and 1 time during the night.

It may take several minutes to empty the bladder completely. Men should sit initially to make sure that the bladder is emptied.

Muscles: Because the neobladder does not expel urine, the abdominal muscles must tighten, and the sphincter muscles relax, so exercises, including Kegel, should be done before surgery.

Incontinence: Some is inevitable; people must be willing and able to catheterize. Some people may never completely empty the bladder and may need to catheterize once or several times a day.

Irrigation: Rarely needed after the immediate post-operative period.

Intubation/Catheterizing the Continent Cutaneous Urinary Diversion

The procedure for intubation/catheterizing the continent cutaneous urinary diversion is explained below:

1. Gather supplies and wash hands.
2. Remove stomal covering.
3. Sit on or near toilet or with a basin beneath stoma.
4. Lubricate end of catheter with water or water-soluble lubricant.
5. Insert catheter into stoma and allow draining by gravity.
6. If catheter plugs or doesn't drain properly, remove the catheter, and rinse it with warm water under the faucet to remove mucus that may be blocking the lumen.
7. When draining is complete, remove catheter.
8. Cleanse peristomal skin and apply a clean stoma covering.
9. Cleanse reusable catheters by washing with soap and hot water; rinse thoroughly, pushing water through the catheter with a syringe.
10. Dry catheters on a paper towel; dry thoroughly inside and out before storing in a Ziploc-type bag.
11. Always keep clean catheters separate from used, and NEVER place catheters on the back of the toilet or counters in public restrooms.

Clean Intermittent Catheterization (CIC) for Males

CIC for males:

1. Gather supplies; wash hands.
2. Sit on toilet or chair with container near.
3. Clean end of penis and urethral opening with soap and water or individually packaged wipes containing benzalkonium chloride.
4. Lubricate catheter with water-soluble lubricant (or water).
5. Hold penis by the sides, perpendicular to the body or pointing slightly upward.
6. Gently insert catheter into meatus, guiding it through the penis. There may be resistance when the catheter passes the prostate. Deep breathing and relaxing may help to advance the catheter. Do not force past a blockage.
7. When urine flow begins, insert the catheter 1 inch more.
8. When drainage ceases, withdraw catheter incrementally, making sure bladder is empty.
9. Wash reusable catheter with soap and hot water. Rinse completely and dry. Store in a clean dry place or carrying case/Ziploc bag. Reusable catheters last about 2-4 weeks, but should be soaked in a white vinegar solution once weekly.

Clean Intermittent Catheterization (CIC) for Females

CIC for females:

1. Gather supplies; wash hands.
2. Sit on toilet or stand with one foot on toilet.
3. Clean vulva and urethral opening with soap and water or individually packaged wipes containing benzalkonium chloride, wiping top to bottom.
4. Lubricate catheter with water-soluble lubricant (or water).
5. Spread labia with second and fourth fingers of one hand; feel for meatus with middle finger.
6. Gently insert catheter into meatus, guiding it upward. Insert 2-3 inches until urine flow; then slowly insert another inch.
7. When drainage ceases, withdraw catheter incrementally, making sure bladder is empty.
8. Wash reusable catheter with soap and hot water. Rinse completely and dry. Store in a clean dry place or carrying case/Ziploc bag. Reusable catheters last about 2-4 weeks, but should be soaked in a white vinegar solution once weekly.
9. Observe urine flow or drain urine into a container and measure if signs of infection or incomplete emptying.

Children Requiring Clean Intermittent Catheterization

The following are special considerations for children requiring clean intermittent catheterization:

- **Age/maturity**: For sense of self-worth and independence, children should become independent in catheterization. Usually, a child needs mental age of 5 and normal physical dexterity to manage catheterization. Most children can catheterize without supervision by the age of 7 or 8.
- **Physical dexterity**: Physical disabilities or lack of dexterity may delay or prevent independent catheterization.
- **Psychological readiness**: Children must be willing to do the procedure. Having the child help at a very young age, such as gathering equipment or holding supplies, can help the child to gain confidence.

- **School**: Children can manage catheterization at school. The teacher, principal, and school nurse or aide should be aware of children's needs. The school nurse or aide can assist. Careful scheduling around breaks will minimize lost class time. If possible, arrange for children to use a private bathroom if available. Make sure that extra supplies are available at school.
- **Latex**: Avoid latex products as allergies may develop.

Metabolic Acidosis and Other Malabsorption Problems

Metabolic acidosis: The normal bladder does not reabsorb fluid or salts from urine, but the intestinal tissue, especially from the colon, used in the creation of the urinary reservoir retains its ability to secrete and absorb ions and fluids, including sodium ions, bicarbonate, and ammonium. This can result in an increase in hydrogen, chloride, and serum urea and creatinine. These problems can occur at any time so people should be monitored for metabolic acidosis. If systemic alkalization is not done, these chronic metabolic disturbances can lead to demineralization of the bones.

Malabsorption: Less transit time leads to diarrhea, malabsorption of bile salts and Vitamin B12 and sometimes fat and fat-soluble vitamins (A, D, E, K), predisposing the person to gallstones, kidney stones, and steatorrhea (fat in feces).

- **Management**: Systemic alkalization is achieved through restriction of chloride intake. Sodium bicarbonate, chlorpromazine, nicotinic acids, and vitamins may be administered.

Urinary Tract Infection, Urinary Retention/Obstruction, and Pouchitis

Urinary tract infection:

- **Urine**: May be cloudy, concentrated, bloody, foul smelling, mucusy, or purulent. May have urinary leakage/incontinence.
- **Pain**: May have flank pain, low back pain, or abdominal cramping.
- **Systemic**: May develop fever with or without chills and a general feeling of malaise and lethargy.
- **Prevention**: Drink 8-10 glasses of liquid, maintain acidity of urine, catheterize on schedule and/or empty bladder completely, and avoid over-distention of reservoir.

Urinary retention/obstruction:

- **Pain**: May have pain in abdomen, lower back, flank, or pelvis.
- **Distention**: May have feeling of abdominal fullness and abdomen may appear distended.
- **Systemic**: Nausea.
- **Prevention**: Catheterize on regular schedule and irrigate as necessary to remove accumulation of mucus in reservoir. Empty bladder completely with each intubation.

Pouchitis:

- **Urine**: Increased mucus and blood urine.
- **Pain**: Pain that may be localized to area of reservoir but may be more generalized.
- **Systemic**: Fever, general malaise.
- **Preventive**: Careful follow-up care and regular monitoring of residual urine volumes.

Postoperative Complications of the Neobladder

The following are postoperative complications of the neobladder:

- **Metabolic acidosis**: Can occur at any time because of reabsorption of fluid or salts through the intestinal tissue of the neobladder and requires systemic alkalization to prevent demineralization of bones.
- **Vitamin B-12 deficiency**: Loss of a portion of the ileum can result in malabsorption.
- **Anastomotic leaks**: Can occur in the pouch or intestines.
- Urinary abnormalities:
    - **Retention**: May be a sign of tumor recurrence, stenosis, or excessive mucus.
    - **Incontinence**: Some incontinence, especially nocturnal enuresis, is common because there is less feeling of bladder fullness. About 10% will have stress incontinence or complete incontinence after procedure.
    - **Calculi**: May be related to persistent bacteriuria. May occur if the bladder is not completely emptied, resulting in urinary stasis, or if urine is exposed to staples or permanent.
    - **Urinary infection**: Recurrent infections and low-grade bacteriuria are common. May have bouts of pyelonephritis.
    - **Fistulas**: Gastrointestinal fistula or ureteral fistulas may occur.
    - **Pouchitis**: Non-specific inflammation of neobladder reservoir.
    - **Stenosis**: Ceco-urethral or ileo-urethral anastomosis stenosis may develop.

Complications Related to Anastomotic Leaks with Creation of Neobladder

The following are complications related to anastomotic leaks with creation of the neobladder:

- **Urinary extravasation**: Urinary leaks may occur from any of the urinary anastomosed areas. Leakage around the sites of the implanted ureters can lead to leakage into the peritoneal cavity.
    - **Symptoms**: Abdominal distension and discomfort as well as urinary leakage around tubes and drains or through the incisions.
    - **Treatment**: Separation of the suture lines may require surgical repair, but surgeons may decide to insert a nephrostomy tube for urinary drainage to allow the suture lines time to heal without urinary pressure. Stents or drainage tubes may be reinserted as well. Intraperitoneal pouch leaks are more difficult to treat medically than extraperitoneal leaks.
- **Fecal leakage**: This is less common than urinary extravasation but can occur at the sites where the fecal section was removed.
    - **Symptoms**: Usually relate to acute peritonitis with fever, chills, abdominal pain, rigidity and distention and an absence of bowel sounds.
    - **Treatment**: Requires antibiotic therapy and immediate surgical intervention.

Special Populations

Side Effects Related to Adjuvant (Postoperative) Chemotherapy

Side effects related to adjuvant (postoperative) chemotherapy for those with ostomies are listed and explained below:

- **Myelosuppression**: People may suffer anemia but depression of the white count is a more serious problem as this compromises the immune system, leaving people susceptible to infection. People must know protective measures, such as avoiding crowds to prevent infections.
- **Mucositis**: Entire mucosa of GI tract can become inflamed, swollen, and painful. Tissue may become infected. Saline mouthwashes, topical anesthetics, and analgesics may help relieve discomfort, promote adequate intake, and prevent infection.
- **Peripheral neuropathies**: Compromised sensation in hands may make ostomy care difficult. Person may need temporary assistance.
- **Skin reactions**: Some drugs may cause photosensitivity so people need to avoid the sun. Hand and foot syndrome can cause severe pain in hands and feet, making self-care difficult.
- **Nausea/vomiting**: Bland foods and anti-emetics may help. Adequate fluid intake is necessary to avoid developing constipation or dehydration. Strong odors, such as food odors or perfume, may trigger nausea.

Side Effects Related to Adjuvant (Postoperative) Radiation for Those with Ostomies

Side effects related to adjuvant (postoperative) radiation for those with ostomies are listed and explained below:

- **Injury to small bowel and rectal area**: Causes diarrhea, often treated with antidiarrheals, such as Lomotil or Imodium, which can in turn cause constipation. Mucosa of bowel becomes denuded. Bland diet with low residue and lactose may relieve symptoms. Stoma may ooze stool frequently and pouches may need to be changed more often.
- **Skin reactions**: May cause pain, burning, dryness, and irritation in radiated tissue. Irritated peristomal tissue may require non-adhesive pouch or skin barrier powder.
- **Fatigue**: People need time to rest and should schedule activities to avoid over-exertion. If fatigue severe, they may need temporary assistance with ostomy or personal care.
- **Nausea/vomiting**: Bland foods and anti-emetics may help. Adequate fluid intake is necessary to avoid developing constipation or dehydration.
- **Proctitis/cystitis**: Organs near radiated area may suffer inflammation and infection, causing pain and complications.
- **Sexual dysfunction**: Males may suffer erectile dysfunction; and females, vaginal stenosis. Open discussion and information about treatment options should be provided.

Urinary Tract Infections in Urostomy Patients

Urinary tract infections are common in urostomy patients and often-chronic low-grade kidney infections develop over time, so observing for urinary infections and treating promptly are very important:

- **Changes in character** of urine:
  - **Appearance**: The urine may become cloudy from mucus or purulent material. Hematuria may be present.
  - **Color**: Urine usually becomes concentrated and may be dark yellow/orange or brownish in color.
  - **Odor**: Urine may have a very strong or foul odor.
  - **Output**: Urinary output may decrease markedly.
- **Pain**: There may be lower back or flank pain from inflammation of the kidneys.
- **Systemic**: Fever, chills, headache, and general malaise often accompany urine infections. Some people suffer lack of appetite as well as nausea and vomiting. Fever usually indicates that the infection has affected the kidneys. Children may develop incontinence or loose stools and cry excessively.
- **Urine specimen**: Specimen should be taken directly from the stoma after the pouch is removed and peristomal skin cleansed.

Collecting Sterile Urine Specimen from Ileal Conduit

Do not collect urine from the bottom of the bag as this is where bacteria will collect and the specimen can give an inaccurate result. Catheterization of the ileal urostomy should be done using aseptic technique. Clean gloves should be worn to remove the ostomy pouch and clean the stoma site with clean water. After the catheterization tray is opened, sterile gloves should be worn. Gently force urine out before inserting the catheter. Lubricate the 14 Fr catheter and insert it about 7 centimeters, or about 2 ¼ inches, into the center of the stoma. If there is resistance, do not force the catheter, but try to rotate it until it slides in easily. Place the end of the catheter into a sterile specimen cup to collect the urine. The patient may need to roll, bear down, or cough to express the urine. Once the specimen is collected, remove the catheter and replace the ostomy pouch. It is important to note on the specimen cup or lab order that the specimen was obtained via an ileal conduit.

SELECTING POUCHING SYSTEMS AND ACCESSORIES FOR NEW OSTOMIES

When selecting a pouching system and accessories, personal choice affects choice but considerations include:

- **Open or closed system**: An open system has a clamp or clip at the bottom that allows the bag to be opened and drained. The open system is most appropriate for those with continuous or liquid drainage, such as an ileostomy. A closed system is appropriate for an ostomy that is more predictable, such as those whose elimination is generally on a regular schedule or those who irrigate and have little or no discharge between irrigations.
- **One- or two-piece systems**: A one-piece system requires the entire appliance be changed each time, which increases the need for supplies and time needed to change the appliance. A two-piece system allows only the outer bag to be replaced as needed.
- **Barriers/wafers**: The type of barrier/wafer that attaches to the skin vary widely with some flat and others convex, so selection may depend on the condition of the stoma and the site. The type of adhesive varies, and some types may be more irritating to skin than others.
- **Accessories**: Various accessories are available, including ostomy belts to help secure the appliance, pouch covers, convex inserts, skin barrier pastes, tapes to secure, and adhesive remover.

Fistula Management

Management

Fistula management typically begins with conservative medical treatment because most close without surgical intervention. Treatment may include broad spectrum antibiotics if the area about the fistula appears infected or if the patient has fistulae associated with Crohn's disease. Infliximab may be administered to patients with Crohn's disease to decrease inflammation and promote healing of fistulae. Containment of drainage is important in order to maintain **perifistular skin** integrity, especially if the drainage contains fecal material, which has enzymes that are destructive of the skin. Continuous suction devices or stoma appliances that provide a skin barrier should be used to protect the perifistular tissue. Perifistular skin should be cleansed with a special cleaning product (such as Cavilon No-Rinse Skin Cleanser) or with tap water and a skin barrier applied. Crusting is a procedure in which a thin layer of ostomy or stoma powder is applied to wet or denuded skin about the fistula and then sprayed with an alcohol-free barrier film to form a protective "crust" to which an appliance can be attached.

Negative Pressure Wound Therapy

Negative pressure wound therapy (NPWT) uses subatmospheric (negative) pressure (-50 to -125 mm HG) with a suction unit and a semi-occlusive vapor-permeable dressing. The suction reduces periwound and interstitial edema, decompresses vessels, improves circulation, and contains effluent. NPWT stimulates production of new cells, decreases colonization of bacteria, increases the rate of granulation and re-epithelialization, reduces wound size, and increases spontaneous closure rates. The wound must be debrided of necrotic tissue prior to treatment. NPWT is contraindicated with wound malignancy, untreated osteomyelitis, exposed blood vessels, unprotected bowel in wound base, and untreated sepsis.

- **Stoma management**: Used for peristomal wound management of separation, skin breakdown, mucocutaneous dehiscence, and open abdomen with stoma.
- **Fistula management**: Used for enterocutaneous fistulae with open wounds, periwound tissue breakdown, containment of high-output effluence, and healing of open complex abdominal wounds.
- **Wound management**: Used for open surgical wounds, pressure injuries, diabetic foot ulcers, dehiscence, grafts/flaps, large cavity wounds, and burns.

Best practices include protecting exposed bowel with non-adherent layers but not applying foam directly to mucosa, using stoma paste and rings to seal edges about high-output fistulae, monitoring output volume and quality, and avoiding excessive negative pressure on bowel by using low-pressure settings.

Octreotide

Octreotide acetate (Mycapssa, Sandostatin, Sandostatin LAR) is a synthetic analog of somatostatin, a peptide hormone that inhibits several GI hormones. Within the GI tract, octreotide inhibits secretion of gastric acid, bile, pancreatic enzymes, and intestinal fluids; suppresses release of serotonin, gastrin, and vasoactive intestinal peptide; and reduces intestinal motility, splanchnic blood flow. Octreotide is available for IM, SQ, PO, or IV administration. When used for wound care, octreotide reduces effluent volume, decreases the risk of skin breakdown, and facilitates granulation. Octreotide is used as adjunctive therapy and is most effective in controlling pancreatic and small bowel (duodenal and high-output jejunal or ileal fistulae) output. Adverse effects can include confusion, dizziness, arrhythmia, bradycardia, blurred vision, hearing loss, abdominal pain, nausea, diarrhea, gallstones, hyperglycemia, hypoglycemia, anemia, arthralgia, myalgia, and alopecia. During administration of octreotide, monitoring should include electrolytes, glucose, fluid balance, output volume, and abdominal imaging to evaluate closure.

Additional Treatment Options

Additional treatment for fistulas include:

- **Antibiotics**: Antibiotics, such as metronidazole, are first line of treatment but often combined with other therapies, such as surgical drainage or excision.
- **Corticosteroids**: Corticosteroids may be used in conjunction with antibiotics and other therapy for Crohn's disease.
- **Drains**: There is evidence that treating abscesses with antibiotics and drainage can prevent fistula formation. Drains/tubes may be left in place to ensure drainage or keep existing fistulas open.
- **Seton**: A suture is placed to hold the fistula open (draining seton). If a fistula heals at the surface and remains open underneath, the discharge will tunnel to the surface again.
- **Autologous fibrin glue**: Glue is used to close fistula.
- **Fistulotomy/fistulectomy**: Excision is often most effective treatment for a fistula. Staged repairs may be done. Surgical treatment may involve open surgery, endoscopic, or laparoscopic approaches. Conservative treatment may precede surgical therapy, but terminal or Crohn's disease patients are poor surgical candidates.

Tube and Drain Management

Securement Techniques for Percutaneous Tubes/Drains

Various types of tubes and drains, such as Penrose, may be inserted into the periwound area in order to collect fluids. The tube/drain may be open—draining directly into absorbent dressings—or closed—drainage collected in a portable suction device, such as the Hemovac or Jackson-Pratt drain. Drains should be secured, often with transparent film or tape at or near the exit site. If a portable suction device or drainage bag is attached to the tube/drain, the tubing should also be secured to the patient's clothing with a safety pin or clip below the operative site, checking to make sure that the tubing is not kinked. Drains may be lightly sutured in place in order to prevent them from inadvertently falling out. In that case, the suture and the tissue about the suture should be examined with each dressing change, but the dressing generally provides the additional securement needed.

Enteral Feeding Tube Complications

Occlusion

Prevention of occlusion involves proper administration of medications and feedings, and maintaining a regular schedule of flushing. Tubes should be flushed with 30 mL of water at least every 4 hours as well as before and after feedings and administration of medications. Medications should be in liquid form or crushed completely and enteric-coated or delayed release preparations should be avoided. Feeding solutions should be liquid consistency. Flushing of occluded tube involves first checking for kinks or obvious problems, attaching a 30-60 mL syringe and aspirating fluid. Then, 5-10 mL of water can be slowly instilled (over about a minute) and aspirated a number of times to try to loosen occlusion. After clamping for 10-15 minutes, the flushing procedure can be repeated with warm water. If the water fails, a multi-enzyme cocktail or pancrease and sodium bicarbonate solution should be attempted. If all flushing fails, the physician should be notified.

Displacement

Displacement of tube is usually the result of inadequate stabilization. Foley catheters must be marked where they exit the stoma to check for migration. Gastrostomy tubes with an internal balloon or mushroom tip, measured markings, and an external disk are easier to stabilize, but internal device should be checked daily by gently pulling until resistance is felt. External stabilizing devices can be applied to the skin to hold the tube in place. The tube may also be taped to the abdomen or secured with a binder. Sometimes surgeons suture the tube in place, especially those with no balloon, such as jejunostomy tubes, which can become easily dislodged. A solid skin barrier with the tube fed through an anchored baby nipple is an inexpensive stabilizer. Position and length of tube should be carefully documented. Balloon volume should be checked weekly to insure there are no leaks. Skin beneath disks/bumpers should be checked frequently.

Skin Irritation and Peristomal Hyperplasia Complications

Skin irritation is caused by gastric secretions or feeding solutions leaking about the tube and making contact with the skin, causing erythema, swelling, pain, and denuded areas. Control leakage can prevent skin irritation. One method is to insert a smaller tube or remove the tube for several hours to shrink the stoma. An ostomy pouching system with skin barrier may be necessary if drainage is measurable and persistent. **Treatment** includes careful cleansing of the peristomal skin and application of a skin barrier. Denuded areas require a skin barrier cream, such as zinc oxide, or skin barrier powder. Alcohol-based barrier wipes should not be used.

Peristomal hyperplasia usually results from irritation caused by latex tubes, tube migration, or moisture. Prevention must involve identifying the causative agent. **Treatment** may include cauterization with silver nitrate sticks, debridement, topical steroid creams (triamcinolone 0.5%), antifungal powder/cream, or diathermy treatments.

Chemical Cauterization of Peristomal Hyperplasia

Peristomal hyperplasia involves an overgrowth of granulation tissue about the stoma of feeding tubes, resulting from irritation, tube migration, or moisture. Often, the etiology is unclear.

Hyperplasia is the result of proliferation of capillaries that form around and inside of the stoma. This tissue may cause pain, bleeding, or oozing is frequently treated with cauterization with silver nitrate sticks. Care must be taken to use silver nitrate only on the granulation tissue as it can cause painful burns if it inadvertently touches other tissue.

Chemical cauterization involves first applying a skin barrier around the tissue to be cauterized. Silver nitrate sticks usually need to be moistened with small amount of sterile water to activate. Apply silver nitrate to tissue by running the tip of the stick in a rolling manner over the tissue to be cauterized. Cauterization is usually required 2 to 3 times weekly until granulation tissue resolves.

Buried Bumper Syndrome Complications

Buried Bumper Syndrome involves migration of the internal bumper into the gastric mucosa. The most common cause is excessive traction pulling the bumper against the gastric mucosa for extended periods, sometimes causing necrotic lesions and abscesses. Small bumpers, stiff bumpers, and malnutrition are also implicated. Symptoms include partial or complete occlusion of the tube, erythema and swelling about stoma as well as pain in the abdominal wall. The bumper may be palpable on examination. Treatment depends upon degree of injury to gastric mucosa. In all cases, the tube must be removed either by external traction or surgical excision with endoscopy. If injury to mucosa is minor, a tube can be reinserted. If there is an extensive necrosis or abscess, healing may take 4 months or longer, and the tube should be inserted in a different site. Prevention requires careful observation and leaving 1.5 cm between the external bumper and the skin to prevent excessive traction.

Preventing and Treating Aspiration and Improper Tube Placement Complications

Aspiration is a common problem that can lead to pneumonia and poses a risk for those with multiple medical problems, such as dysphagia, decreased level of alertness, previous episodes of pneumonia or ileus. Large-bore tubes and mechanical ventilators have also been implicated. Prevention includes using a small-bore feeding tube, checking residuals every 4-6 hours, holding feedings if residual is greater than 100-150 mL, Elevating the head of the bed to 30-45 degrees, and using continuous feeding rather than bolus. Treatment may require a jejunal extension tube or replacement of gastrostomy with jejunostomy.

Improper tube placement is the result of lack of proper prevention efforts prior to tube placement. Gastrostomy tubes are usually placed in the left upper quadrant, but should avoid folds or creases that might cause leakage. General guidelines include placing the tube 3-5 cm below the costal margin. Treatment may include using skin barriers or pouching systems. In worst cases, replacement may be considered.

Important Terms

Contrast Enema: Contrast liquid, usually barium, instilled rectally to outline inside of intestines, followed by x-rays of abdomen.

Endoscopy: Procedure for minimally invasive surgical techniques using an instrument with rigid or flexible tube that can be inserted into the body, usually through an orifice or incision, to visually inspect, photograph, take biopsies, do surgical procedures, and remove foreign objects.

Intravenous Pyelogram: Imaging technique where intravenous contrast dye is given to highlight urinary structures on x-ray. Used to show path and rate of urinary flow through urinary tract.

Ultrasound: Imaging technique using high-frequency sound waves to create computer images of vessels, tissues, and organs. Used to view organs, evaluate function, and assess circulation.

Voiding Cystourethrogram (VCUG): Catheter is inserted through urethra into bladder, which is filled with liquid containing contrast dye. X-rays are taken as the bladder fills and empties, showing function and reverse flow of urine to ureters and kidneys.

Appendicostomy: Appendix brought to abdominal wall to form a stoma, usually at umbilicus, to provide open channel for insertion of catheter to irrigate bowel to prevent constipation. Procedure may be done to relieve constipation in those with myelomeningocele.

Clean Intermittent Catheterization (CIC): Procedure in which a straight catheter is inserted into the opening to the bladder, usually the urethra, to empty the bladder completely. It may be done intermittently as a temporary procedure or for long-term management of the bladder.

Cystoplasty: Surgical repair of defect in bladder. May be done as reductive procedure to reduce large distended bladder or to correct other defects.

Pyeloplasty: Incision into and repair of kidney pelvis.

Ureterostomy: The ureter is opened to abdominal wall with a stoma as a urinary diversion.

Vesicostomy: Bladder mucosa opened to lower abdominal wall with creation of stoma to allow for permanent or temporary urinary diversion.

Care Planning

Principles of Patient-Centered Care

Supporting Patient and Caregiver Goals

Preventive goals: Measures to prevent disease/disability or prevent deterioration or complications of existing disorder. May include screening (BP, Pap smear, mammograms, blood glucose), disease education, fall prevention, smoking cessation, substance abuse rehabilitation, vaccinations, nutritional counseling, and exercise.

Maintenance goals: Measures to control existing disorder in order to maintain status. May include therapy (OT, PT, ST), education, ongoing lifestyle changes, supervision, ongoing assessment, medications, blood glucose management, and treatment. Maintenance therapy may follow primary therapy for some diseases, such as cancer, in order to maintain status.

Curative goals: Measures intended to cure disease rather than simply to alleviate symptoms or pain. May include medications, casting (as for broken limbs), radiotherapy, dialysis, transfusions, chemotherapy, physical therapy, rehabilitation therapy, and surgical interventions. Note: Curative treatments are also sometimes used for palliation but without intent to cure.

Access to Care

A number of factors may affect **access to care**:

- **Proximity to medical services**: Some geographic areas have more medical services than others. For example, some rural areas lack both hospitals and physicians. Cutting edge treatments may be unavailable in some areas.
- **Socioeconomic status**: Lack of insurance or money to pay for medical services prevents many people from seeking medical care or complying with treatments. Many cannot afford to pay for prescription drugs or supplies.
- **Language differences**: Non-English speakers may not be able to communicate needs or to understand information, such as the treatment plan.
- **Health literacy**: Some may have little knowledge and understanding of anatomy, physiology, disease, and medical treatments.
- **Disability status**: Disabilities may have a profound effect of access to care or very little, depending on the type of disability and the resources available, but some disabilities impair mobility and the ability to access care.
- **Transportation**: Private and public transportation may be unavailable or the cost prohibitive.
- **Race and ethnicity**: Inequalities faced by minority populations often extend to medical services. Many live in poor neighborhoods that provide little access to medical services.

Goals of Rehabilitation for Ostomy Patients

Goals of rehabilitation include the following:

- **Independence**: Person should be able to do as much self-care as possible, with accommodations for disabilities or limitations.
- **Stoma care**: Person should be aware of complications, including signs and symptoms and should understand how to prevent complications and deal with them effectively and know when to seek medical attention.
- **Peristomal care**: Person should understand importance of regular assessment of skin and know how to avoid irritation and treat irritation if it should arise.
- **Pouching**: Person should know pouching options and how to apply, use, clean, and change pouches.
- **Ostomy function**: Person should understand normal functioning and be aware of changes that need attention or could be a sign of complications. Person should be able to irrigate if necessary.
- **Support system**: Person should be aware of support groups and agencies/organizations that provide information and should identify family and friends who can be of assistance.

Active Listening

Active listening requires more than simply hearing what another individual is saying. Active listening includes observing the other individual carefully for nonverbal behaviors, such as posture, eye contact, and facial expression, as well as understanding and reflecting on what the person is saying. The listener should observe carefully for inconsistencies in what the individual is saying or comments that require clarification. Feedback is critical to active listening because it shows the speaker that one is paying attention and showing interest and respect. Feedback may be as simple as nodding the head in agreement but should also include asking questions or making comments to show full engagement. Listening with empathy is especially important because it helps to build a connection with the speaker. The listener should communicate empathy with words: "You feel (emotion) because (experience)," because the speaker may not be sensitive to what the listener is comprehending.

Special Considerations

Counseling on Intimacy for Those with Ostomies

Emotional element validates person's anxieties and encourages expression. Sexual desire and activity can alter after surgery and affect the body image and sense of well-being and attractiveness. Provide support for both patient and partner, whose response to the ostomy can have a profound effect on the patient.

Physical element involves discussion of physical changes that may affect sexual functioning and alternative means of sexual activity. Discuss physical limitations and pain and how they relate to sexual activity. Encourage experimentation to find sexual expression rewarding to both partners.

Educational element provides practical information, such as the importance of emptying the pouch prior to sexual activity. Using smaller, low-profile pouching systems, or specially designed undergarments may help a person feel more comfortable. Pamphlets and information about sexual activity should be provided to patient.

Communicative element encourages both patient and partner to discuss fears and feelings about sexual activity. Open and honest communication is critical.

PLISSIT Model for Communicating About Sexuality

PLISSIT model (developed by Annon in the 1970s and still applicable in the clinical environment) for communicating about sexuality is explained below:

- Level one:
  - **Permission**: Gives the person permission to have feelings or attitudes and to do or not do something. Reassure person feelings are not abnormal. Pointing out consequences of choices is important to put patient's choices in perspective. Attempt to establish open communication by helping person to feel comfortable.
- Level two:
  - **Limited Information**: Information should help to dispel misconceptions and fears and should be specifically related to needs and concerns of patient. Information should be factual about the effects of surgery on sexuality.
- Level three:
  - **Specific Suggestions**: At this point, the person needs to take action or seek treatment with medical guidance. Some specific suggestions might include the use of lubricants, emptying pouch before sexual activity, or using pouch covers.
- Level four:
  - **Intensive Therapy**: This involves referral to an appropriate specialist as the person may, for example, need reconstructive surgery or psychotherapy beyond what the nurse is able to provide.

Supporting Patients Through Body Image Issues After Placement of an Ostomy

Ostomy patients often develop negative body images even though their quality of life may have improved. Some may become depressed and withdrawn or even suicidal, and others may exhibit anger. Patients may go through a number of phases on the path to psychological acceptance: panic/shock, denial, acknowledgement, and acceptance. Patients may have concerns about sexuality. The nurse should practice active listening and encourage patients to express feelings and describe what is most concerning to them, such as the fear of leaks or odors, and help patients to find solutions to those concerns to give them a feeling of control. The patient may benefit from guidance about clothing options and different types of appliances as well as ostomy management and support services that are available. Actively engaging the patient in care of the ostomy can help the patient to become more accepting and confident. The patient may also benefit from assistance and practice in briefly describing or explaining the surgery to family and friends because patients often feel embarrassment or shame.

Supporting Patients with Disabilities

Patients often face functional, emotional, and psychosocial challenges in dealing with ostomies, diversions, and draining wounds. Special considerations must be made for patients with additional **disabilities**. These patients may need adaptive devices, such as pouching aids and mirror stands, and pouching and skin care may need to be done in seated position. If patients have a one-sided weakness or paralysis, procedures may need to be simplified or broken into short sessions. If patients are visually impaired, they may need tactile labels, verbal cues, and high-contrast materials. For cognitive impairment, step-by-step visual aids may help, and caregivers may need training.

Terminal Care Issues for Those with Ostomies

Terminal care issues for those with ostomies include the following:

- **Curative vs. palliative**: Curative and palliative care are not mutually exclusive. Palliative care can begin during curative care to help patient and family plan and to provide services they will need to cope. The goal of palliative care is to provide the best quality of life possible.
- **Pain control**: By law, adequate pain control is the right of the terminal patient. Discussing different methods of pain control reassures the terminal patient.
- **Hospice care**: Hospice resources are invaluable to patient and caregivers, providing supplies, assistance, and respite.
- **Self-determination**: Patients have the right to self-determination regarding their care. Patients should be encouraged to complete an Advance Directive outlining their wishes.
- **Ostomy care**: Plans should be made early regarding care of the ostomy if patient unable to do so. This may entail training caregivers or making arrangements for Home Health care. Discussions about diet/fluids/constipation/diarrhea and how to manage these issues are necessary.

Additional Considerations

Neonates

There are important considerations regarding ostomies for neonates. Most ostomies are performed for necrotizing enterocolitis, so the infant is often critically ill. Other indications include meconium ileus, intestinal atresia, Hirschsprung disease, and anorectal abnormalities. For ileostomy/colostomy, stool production is limited for the first one to two days, so petrolatum gauze is applied to protect the stoma but a bag is generally not applied. Because skin is friable, especially in preterm neonates, adhesive and skin sealant use should be limited, and adhesive remover should be avoided with adhesive loosened with a cloth dampened with warm water. Peristomal skin should be cleansed only with water or, if necessary, pH neutral soap, which is thoroughly rinsed. No skin sealant containing alcohol should be used. Likewise, skin barrier pastes should be avoided because of alcohol content, although a low-alcohol paste may be used if necessary to secure an appliance. Only appliances intended for neonates should be used. Appliances are available in various sizes and shapes. Gas production is often increased with neonates because of crying, so pouches should have a charcoal filter that allows release of gas.

Pediatric Patients

The following are care plan issues of long-term management of conventional colostomies in pediatric patients:

- **Activity/exercise**: Can engage in almost all activities/exercises, but should avoid rough contact sports and heavy lifting.
- **Clothing**: Should provide easy access to pouch, so children can manage care. Infants and small children may need one-piece outfits to prevent them from removing pouch.
- **Food/fluids**: Should be taught types of foods/fluids to avoid and good eating habits.
- **Bathing**: Can bathe/shower with or without a pouch. If frequent fecal leakage, a pouch can be worn during the bath.
- **Travel**: Should carry ostomy supplies for the entire trip as they may be hard to find and carry an adequate supply in carry-on luggage if flying.
- **School**: The school nurse, principal, and teacher should be aware of the child's colostomy and extra supplies and clothing should be available at school.
- **Ostomy supplies**: Can use closed-end pouches to avoid emptying appliance at school or special events. Ostomy belts and pouch covers may provide added security.

Obstetrics

Pregnancy in Women with Ostomies

Implications of pregnancy in women with ostomies are as follows:

- **Nausea**: Maintain adequate fluid intake to prevent constipation/obstruction.
- **Stoma**: As abdomen becomes larger, stoma may enlarge and change shape, becoming more oval. It may recede or prolapse. Measure frequently. Stoma usually returns to normal after delivery.
- **Vaginal delivery**: If there is scar tissue from removal of the rectum, an episiotomy may be necessary. Some may not be suitable candidates for vaginal delivery. Pressure during delivery often expresses stool, so appliance should be changed after delivery. As girth increases, women may need to use a mirror to view stoma.
- **Ultrasounds**: Appliances can loosen because of oil used during procedure, so clean abdomen thoroughly and change appliance after procedure. The absence of a bladder in some women may complicate viewing and the position of the stoma may interfere with viewing of the fetus.
- **Breast-feeding**: There are usually no contraindications unless the medications the woman is taking are passed into the breast milk and considered unsafe for the child.

Ileostomy Care During Pregnancy

Implications of ileostomy care during pregnancy are as follows:

- **Timing pregnancy**: If the ileostomy is for inflammatory bowel disease, it's better to be pregnant during inactive periods of disease as active disease may lead to miscarriage or premature birth. However, about 1/3 of women with inflammatory bowel disease become active during the pregnancy and receive medical treatment during pregnancy.
- **Ileostomy care**: Ileostomy may be more active during the pregnancy because of increasing pressure. As the abdomen becomes larger, the stoma often also enlarges and changes shape, becoming more oval. Measure from time to time and change sizes as necessary. Stoma usually returns to normal shortly after delivery.
- **Complications**: There is a slight chance of blockage as the fetus grows and applies pressure. Abdomen may become painful and distended. Liquid diet and rest usually suffice; intravenous fluids may be needed to rest the intestines, so close monitoring of ileostomy functioning is important.
- **Birth**: Vaginal births are possible: some need Cesareans.

Birth Control Issues for Women with Ostomies

Birth control medications: Because of absorption issues, pills may not be suitable for some women with ileostomies, depending upon how much small intestine remains. A higher dose than normal may be needed. With Crohn's disease, absorption may be so compromised that birth control pills are not effective. Injectable progesterone has been used successfully.

Intrauterine device: Generally, the IUD is not advised for women who have never had children, and is not suitable for some with ostomies, especially if uterus is fixed in a different position from usual. Fitting the coil can be a difficult.

Cervical caps/diaphragms: Some can successfully use caps or diaphragms, but if the anatomy of the uterus or vagina was altered, insertion and retention may be problematic.

Condoms: Condoms can be effective birth control if used properly and consistently.

Vasectomy: If it is important to permanently avoid pregnancy, a vasectomy for the male partner may be advisable.

Bariatric

There are important considerations regarding ostomies for obese patients (BMI > 35). The placement of the stoma may pose problems because of abdominal rolls, which must be avoided. The stoma should be placed if possible where it is 5 to 10 cm away from creases and folds and away from the belt line. Because subcutaneous fat may shift, the stoma site should be selected by assessing the patient in both sitting and standing position. Patients with very large breasts and protruding abdomens may have difficulty both visualizing the stoma, especially if it is placed low on the abdomen, and managing appliances. Postoperatively, bariatric patients are more likely to develop stoma necrosis because of impaired circulation. Overweight patients are especially at risk of atelectasis so they must be encouraged to practice deep breathing and coughing and early mobilization is essential. Patients may be able to manage a one-piece pouch better than one with a detachable bag if their abdomens are large. Patients who have also had bariatric surgery to lose weight and then regain the weight may develop an enlarged stoma.

Education and Referral

Principles of Education

Cognitive, Affective, and Psychomotor Learning Abilities

Cognitive ability involves learning and gaining intellectual skills. There are 6 categories to master for effective learning, in order: knowledge, comprehension, application, analysis, synthesis, and evaluation.

Affective ability involves recognizing 5 categories of feelings and values, from simple to complex and is slower to achieve than cognitive learning.

- **Receiving phenomena**: Viewing stoma, accepting need to learn.
- **Responding to phenomena**: Taking active part in care.
- **Valuing**: Understanding value of becoming independent in care.
- **Organizing values**: Understanding how surgery has improved life.
- **Internalizing values**: Accepting condition as part of life, being consistent and self-reliant.

Psychomotor ability involves mastering 7 categories of motor skills necessary for independence, from simple to complex:

- **Perception**: Uses sensory information to learn tasks.
- **Set**: Shows willingness to perform tasks.
- **Guided response**: Follows directions.
- **Mechanism**: Does specific tasks.
- **Complex overt response**: Displays competence in self-care.
- **Adaptation**: Modifies procedures as needed.
- **Origination**: Creatively deals with problems.

Effects of Successive Stages of Cognitive Learning on Teaching

The effects of successive stages of cognitive learning on teaching are as follows:

- Knowledge:
  - Ask for feedback about teaching points.
  - Ask learner to identify equipment, list procedure steps and explain.
- Comprehension:
  - Ask learner to explain principles or procedures in own words: Why are things done this way?
  - Ask learner to summarize purpose of procedures.
- Application:
  - Ask learner to solve problems in different situations: What would happen if...? Or how could this problem be solved?
  - Ask learner to demonstrate procedures.
- Analysis:
  - Question learner to determine ability to distinguish fact from inference: What can happen if the opening is too large in the pouch?
  - Ask learner to troubleshoot: How do you deal with pouch leakage?
- Synthesis:
  - Ask learner to integrate knowledge to solve problems: How can odor issues be resolved?
- Evaluating knowledge:
  - Ask learner questions that demonstrate knowledge by explaining or interpreting: Why is measuring of stoma important?
  - Ask learner to choose the most effective solution to problems.

Effects of Developmental Stage of Learner on Teaching

The effects of developmental stage of learner on teaching are discussed below:

- **Infant/toddler**: Caregivers provide care; instruction encourages bonding and acceptance.
- **Early childhood**: Children learn by participation, such as role-playing, simple explanation, and teaching dolls. Children should be independent in emptying pouch by kindergarten.
- **Childhood**: By age 6, children should be independent in care at school, but ostomy supplies should be at school and school nurse knowledgeable about ostomy care. Child should be completely independent in care by 6th grade. Parents and child should be taught together.
- **Adolescence/young adulthood**: The adolescent may be angry and resistive, extra time and guidance, including visits with other ostomy patients, may help. Parents should allow adolescent to be independent in care.
- **Middle-aged adult**: Adults may have fears about loss of income, status, sexuality, so individualized teaching that includes partners helps them to deal with these issues.
- **Elderly**: Elderly may face physiological and psychological changes. Teaching should provide coping skills and information in stages to avoid overwhelming them.

Health Literacy

Health literacy is the ability to obtain, understand, and consent to medical care, making informed healthcare decisions and must be considered when developing activities. Health literacy includes:

- Reading with comprehension, applying reason to context.
- Understanding graphs and other visual representations of information.
- Using the computer to obtain information.
- Understanding the results of laboratory/radiographic studies.
- Understanding and using basic mathematical computations.
- Articulating concerns and questions.
- Understanding basic anatomy and physiology.
- Having basic knowledge of disease.
- Understanding preventive health measures.
- Knowing how to access health care and health information.

Health literacy may be impacted by a number of factors, including lack of adequate education (low reading level), illiteracy, dementia, and learning disabilities. Those most vulnerable include the elderly, ethnic minorities, immigrants, and those with low income and/or chronic medical or physical health problems. The nurse must evaluate the patient/caregiver to determine their level of health literacy and gear education to that level.

Preoperative and Postoperative Education

Elements of Preoperative Teaching

Elements of preoperative teaching are as follows:

- **Anatomy and physiology**: Should provide information about the gastrointestinal/urinary systems, including basic anatomy and physiology. Explain changes in function after surgery and explain how stoma will redirect fecal material or urine.
- **Stoma**: Should prepare person for mucoid appearance of stoma and explain that stoma lacks sensation so person will not feel need to pass stool/urine and thus the necessity of the pouch. Should discuss initial swelling and appearance of stoma and length of time before edema recedes.
- **Pouching concerns**: Should explain that pouching systems are odor-proof and that gas and odor can be further controlled by attention to diet. Should reassure person that pouching will be easily concealed under clothing.
- **Preoperative preparation**: Should explain all necessary preoperative bowel preparation and diet restrictions so that the bowel is adequately evacuated prior to surgery.
- **Postoperative complication**: Should explain all possible postoperative complications and answer any questions that the person may have about complications.

Preoperative Counseling for Neobladder

The following are elements of preoperative counseling for those planning to have a neobladder:

- **Surgical procedure**: Detailed explanation of the procedure itself, drains, and post-operative care and expectations. If lesion is cancerous, the need for flexibility must be stressed as it may be more difficult to determine the exact surgical procedure in advance.
- **Exercises**: Kegel exercises to strengthen the muscles of the pelvic floor and well as exercises to tighten and relax the sphincter should begin prior to surgery.
- **Urinary care**: Instruction for intermittent self-catheterization should be done prior to surgery. The importance of emptying the bladder and maintenance of a schedule for urination must be stressed.
- **Dietary modifications**: Explanation of the need for fluids and foods to maintain urinary output and help avoid metabolic acidosis and diarrhea.
- **Complications**: Understanding the signs of metabolic acidosis and other complications is important.
- **Bowel care**: Loss of the ileocecal valve and part of the ileum can result in increased diarrhea, so dietary management of bowels is necessary.

Dietary Guidelines for First 6 Weeks After Ostomy Related to Bowel Surgery

Post-surgical swelling in the first 6 weeks after surgery causes the intestinal lumen to narrow, so **dietary modifications** are necessary to prevent obstruction:

- Ensure diet is well balanced and nutritious with at least a minimum of servings from each of the main food groups:
    - 2-3 servings of dairy products
    - 2-3 servings of protein (meats, fish, beans, eggs, & nuts)
    - 6-11 servings of breads and cereal
    - 2-4 servings of fruits
    - 3-5 servings of vegetables
- Avoid high fiber foods, which can cause obstruction.
- Eat 5-6 small meals a day, rather than 3 large meals.
- Introduce one new food at a time and evaluate response to food.
- Chew all foods thoroughly to begin digestive process.
- Cook foods until they are well cooked and tender.
- Drink 8 glasses of fluid each day and avoid using straw, which can cause gas.
- Drink caffeinated beverages in moderation as they can lead to dehydration.

Perianal Skin Care for Ileal Pouch Anal Anastomosis

After ileostomy closure, there may be seepage of fecal material and mucus from the anus, especially at night. The combination of moisture and friction from walking or wiping the area with tissue can cause severe irritation.

- **Avoid anal irritants**: Raw fruits, raw vegetables, oriental vegetables, coconut, dried fruits, spicy foods, seeds, and nuts or other foods (may be individual).
- **Careful cleansing**: Rinse the perineal area with warm water using a squirt bottle or bulb syringe or gently wipe with cotton balls, Tucks, or baby wipes. Avoid washcloths, which are too rough. Avoid soap, which may irritate because of alkalinity. Pat dry, fan, or use cool hair dryer.
- **Preventive skin care**: Apply protective skin barrier cream/ointment—A&D Ointment, Vaseline, or Desitin—in the perianal area. A soft dressing, such as a strip of cotton or a gauze dressing, may be positioned between the buttocks.
- **Clothing**: Wear cotton underwear; avoid synthetic material or restrictive clothes.

Protecting Skin from Fistula Drainage

Providing **skin protection** is critical. Low output fistulas may need only skin barriers and easily-changed absorbent dressings. Creases, folds, and depressions may need to be filled with skin barrier paste, wafers, or powder before solid barriers applied. Solid barriers last as long as they remain intact; Liquid skin sealants, up to 24 hours; Skin powders/pastes, to 24 hours.

Containing drainage is necessary. If drainage cannot be contained with an absorbent dressing, then ostomy appliances with solid skin barriers and pouches are indicated. The barrier should extend at least 1.5 inches around perimeter of fistula. The barrier must adhere to even skin to avoid drainage getting under the barrier, so the opening may need to be enlarged. Pouching systems with barriers that can be cut to fit usually work best. If drainage is extensive, a bedside drainage bag may be used. Very large wounds (more than 4 inches) may require a custom pouching system.

Postoperative Education for Ostomy Patients

Postoperative education for ostomy patients includes:

- **Pouching**: Patients need to know the types of pouching systems available (open/closed, one-piece/two-piece) and should be able to see and manipulate them to determine what they can easily handle and prefer. They must have adequate practice under supervision applying, emptying, and changing the pouching system and must understand how to assess the stoma and surrounding skin each time. Because the stoma may change in size over time, if they are using a cut-to-fit barrier, then patients must learn how to measure the stoma. They also need to understand the frequency of pouch changes.
- **Peristomal skin health**: Patients must learn how to examine, cleanse, and protect peristomal skin and need learn how to recognize and treat problems, such as skin irritation/maceration, burning, itching, odor. They must learn about crusting and various types of skin barriers and fillers, depending on their individual needs.

Educating Patients on Optimal Management

Pelvic Floor Exercises

The pelvic floor muscles cross the floor of the pelvis and attach to the pubic bone and coccyx. The urethra, rectum, and vagina all open through the pelvic floor muscles, which support the pelvic organs.

Caution: Avoid holding the breath or tightening the abdominal or buttocks muscles during pelvic floor exercises.

Procedure: Tighten and squeeze the muscles about the rectum, vagina, and urethra and try to "lift" them inside as though trying to stop from passing gas and urine. Hold. Relax. Rest a few seconds. Repeat.

Schedule: Exercises should be done at least 3 times daily. They may be done while lying down in the morning and evening and while sitting midday.

- **1-2 weeks**: Tighten 1 second, relax 5. Repeat 10 times. Then tighten 5 seconds and relax 10. Repeat 10 times.
- **3-4 weeks**: Tighten 5-10 seconds and relax 10. Repeat 20 times.
- **5-6 weeks**: Tighten 8-10 seconds and relax 10. Repeat 20 times.

Patient Education for Wound Management

Infection Control, Repositioning, and Trauma Avoidance

Infection control: Topics include the importance of hand hygiene, methods for disposal of soiled materials, the risk of healthcare-associated infections (including asking healthcare providers to wash hands), appropriate use of antibiotics, and appropriate wound care.

Repositioning: The need for repositioning, the manner, positions, and frequency vary depending on the patient's condition, but the patient should be apprised of the importance of repositioning to prevent skin breakdown and shown how to reposition, encouraging the patient to reposition at least every 2 hours.

Trauma avoidance: Topics include fall prevention and safe driving as well as measures to improve home safety, such as removal of throw rugs and clutter, improved lighting, installation of handrails and safety bars, and use of shower chairs. Some patients may need information about avoiding choking, fire safety, and safe use of tools (such as knives and clippers).

Tobacco Cessation

Smoking releases carbon monoxide and hydrogen cyanide in the blood and interferes with the delivery of oxygen to the tissues, and nicotine is a vasoconstrictor, resulting in slowed healing. Smoking also increases platelet clumping, increasing risk of clotting. Patients should learn about the effects of smoking on healing and should be provided tobacco cessation aids. A number of medical treatments can assist patients through the withdrawal period, during which the person may experience anxiety, irritability, and nicotine craving. Many of the of the medications contain nicotine, but it is released in a slower manner to avoid the sudden increase in nicotine ("rush") associated with smoking: Nicotine patch, nicotine inhaler, nicotine gum, nicotine lozenge, and nicotine nasal spray. Prescription medications that are taken before quitting and then for up to 6 months include bupropion SR and varenicline. Smoking cessation programs include support groups, online forums (StopSmokingCenter.net) and informational websites (Smokefree.gov). The HHS recommends the 5A program: Ask, advise, assess, assist, and arrange followup.

Issues Related to Caregivers to Optimize Patient's Adaptation and Self- Care

The following are issues related to caregivers to optimize patient's adaptation and self- care:

- **Paid vs. family/friends**: Paid caregivers may or may not have prior training with ostomies but will generally expect to assist with this care. Family or friends may be motivated to help or may be resentful and uncooperative. Identifying a caregiver even for the self-sufficient should be done before a need arises.
- **Knowledge**: Assessing caregiver's knowledge and ability to learn is part of the care plan. Training may need to be modified or done in small steps for some caregivers. Training of the patient and caregiver at the same time is ideal, and can provide an opportunity to discuss the impact the ostomy has on the relationship.
- **Fear/disapproval**: Caregivers who express fear, disgust, or disapproval regarding the ostomy can have a negative impact on the patient and interfere with that person's learning. Acknowledging negative feelings and openly discussing them can often lead to a positive outcome. Alternative care providers may be necessary.

Supply and Information Resources

Information Patients Need to Resume Optimal Lifestyle

The following is general information the patient needs to resume an optimal lifestyle:

- **Ostomy supplies**: Person needs complete list of supplies, supply numbers, and information about billing insurance or Medicare. If necessary, written prescription should be supplied and lists of local, mail order, and online suppliers. Indigent people may need referral to social services for assistance.
- **Dietary information**: Person needs information about foods to avoid, especially in first few weeks after surgery. Person should receive a list of foods that thicken or loosen stool and that cause gas or odor. Urostomy patients should be advised that asparagus, fish, and some spices cause urine odor.
- **Gas/odor management**: Person should learn common causes of gas and odor, which may include smoking, chewing gum, and swallowing air when sleeping or using a straw. Person needs help to assess individual's dietary practices that cause gas/odor. Simethicone with meals and pouch deodorants help reduce odor.
- **Contact/support information**: Person needs to know whom to call or where to go for help or support.

Community and Internet Resources for Patients and Families

The following are types of community and internet resources that patients and their families need to know about:

- **Local agencies**: Local branches of national organizations or local agencies developed to meet particular needs may be available. Senior citizen groups may provide support and information or direct to other resources.
- **Support groups**: Agencies, hospitals, charitable foundations, hospices, and senior citizens groups are just a few that may have support groups for patients and/or caregivers. Attending a support group where patients or caregivers can meet and talk with others facing similar challenges can be very helpful from a practical as well as emotional perspective.
- **Consumer organizations**: Societies, foundations, and associations dedicated to a particular type of health problem or need can be a wealth of information, providing literature, updates on drugs and treatments, and online chat groups or message boards.
- **Product manufacturers/suppliers**: Patients should be aware of local distributors/retailers of ostomy supplies and catalog and Internet resources. In some areas, people may not have ready access to needed supplies.

Resources for Patients

Resources available to the patient include:

- **Support and advocacy**: Support groups are available through many medical centers and hospitals as well as online. Many are sponsored by national organizations and are generally free of cost and available to patients and/or families. National organizations also often provide information about clinical trials and current research.
- **Access to supplies**: Many manufacturers provides assistance programs for those unable to afford supplies, such as dressings, and some national organizations may also provide assistance. Some patients may be eligible for Medicaid, which will cover the costs of necessary supplies and equipment.
- **Post-acute care**: This level of care is less intense than that provided by an acute hospital. Post-acute care may be provided after acute hospitalization or instead of acute hospitalization. Medical treatments can be continued with post-acute care but the focus is more commonly on rehabilitation.

Ostomy, Fistula, and Tube Management

Management Principles for Patient Teaching About Pouching and/or Containment Strategies

Assess patient readiness and ability to learn and manage own care. Provide emotional support and allow person to express feelings.

Consider special needs as those with special needs, such as limited cognitive or physical ability, may need modifications or assistance. People who are hard of hearing, vision-impaired, or illiterate may need video or audiotapes or illustrated instructions.

Do **step-by-step instruction** of main tasks and begin with simple steps such as draining and clamping pouch and continue until person has mastered the main tasks: emptying the pouch, removing the pouch, cleansing and caring for the skin, measuring the stoma, applying a new pouch, and disposing of the old pouch.

Do **on-going assessment** over time and evaluate person's ability to manage pouching while in the hospital, after returning home, and then after one month at home and three months at home to ensure that all questions are answered and problems have been resolved.

Barriers to Self-Care of Pouching and Containment Strategies

The following are psychological, physical, and cognitive barriers to self-care of pouching and containment strategies:

- Psychological barriers:
  - **Emotional instability** may interfere with ability to learn and manage care.
  - **Sexuality issues** may cause people to be anxious about body image, sexual dysfunction, and sexual activity with a stoma appliance. Homosexual patients may need special counseling.
- Physical barriers:
  - **Vision impairment** requires that people wear glasses or any other modifiers in good light. Those who are legally blind need a tactile approach to teaching so that they can use their sense of touch. Braille text or 3-dimensional models may be helpful.
  - **Hearing impairment** requires a quiet environment or translator. Nurse should face patient to facilitate lip reading and use picture diagrams or videos.
  - **Allergies** mean require people to try different system to determine sensitivities or use non-adhesive or modified systems.
  - **Motor impairment** may necessitate simplified ostomy care and consultation with occupational therapist.
- Cognitive Barriers:
  - **Mental acuity** varies, and some may not be able to be independent in care or may need repeated step-by-step instruction over prolonged period of time.

Care Plan Issues of Long-Term Management of Conventional Colostomies

The following are care plan issues of long-term management of conventional colostomies:

- **Work**: Working should pose no special problems unless it involves heavy lifting or digging, which may require a special support to prevent herniation. An ostomy belt can keep the ostomy in place for those whose jobs are very active. Extra supplies and clean clothes should be kept at the workplace, in the car, or in an easily accessible place.
- **Exercise**: An exercise program should be planned with the healthcare provider and should start slowly. For contact sports, a special support or cover for the colostomy can protect the stoma. Always empty the pouch before sports activities, especially swimming. Do not remove the pouch while swimming and secure the edges with waterproof tape.
- **Travel**: Ostomy supplies may not be available in some areas, so carry all supplies needed, including an adequate supply in carry-on bag. Keep supplies in the coolest area of the car so supplies don't melt in hot weather.
- **Bathing**: Pouch may be worn for bathing if likelihood of fecal leakage, but a shower can be taken with or without the pouch as the water will not damage the stoma and leakage will wash down the drain.
- **Relationships**: Open communication and discussion can help relieve anxiety for ostomy patient and others. The dependency involved in ostomy care can cause conflict, and this needs to be addressed.
- **Sex**: Sexual function may be impaired; information about sexual activity and alternate means of sexual expression should be provided. Pouch covers or special underwear can be utilized.
- **Constipation/irrigation**: Management strategies for constipation, prevention of impaction and irrigation should be understood. Adequate fluids, exercise, and fiber intake can help to relieve constipation.
- **Diarrhea**: People with history of diarrhea can use customary methods of control, including adequate fiber, increased carbohydrates, and sufficient fluids. An increase in diarrhea along with symptoms such as dehydration or cramping should be reported to physician.

Multidisciplinary Care Collaboration

Educating Health Care Providers on Ostomy Care Principles

The ostomy care nurse's role in **educating health care providers** on ostomy care includes sharing principles of ostomy care:

- Understanding that initial pouching requirements in the postoperative period may differ from maintenance requirements and usually begin with clear, drainable, cut-to-fit pouches without convexity wafers until healing takes place.
- Helping the patient to achieve a pouching system that improves the patient's quality of life and one that the patient can manage effectively.
- Achieving a predictable wear time, usually at least 3 days but no longer than 7, so ensuring that the appropriate barrier/wafer and appliance is utilized.
- Maintaining peristomal skin in optimal condition and recognizing indications of skin irritation or problems and understanding solutions.
- Helping the patient to deal emotionally with changes in body image related to the ostomy.
- Ensuring that the patient is aware of resources available for supplies/equipment and supportive services, such as support groups and online forums.

Consulting Infectious Disease and Dermatology

The nurse has an essential role in preventing and identifying infection and dermatologic issues and making appropriate **consultations**:

- **Infectious disease**: Referral may be indicated if the patient exhibits a persistent or recurrent local infection or has systemic indications, such as elevated temperature, leukocytosis, and/or sepsis. Careful supervision is often needed to prevent and treat multi-resistant organisms. Patients who are immunocompromised (chemotherapy, transplants, HIV/AIDS) may need monitoring by an infectious disease professional. Referral is often needed for urinary diversions if UTIs are occurring and for infections related to fistulae and percutaneous tubes and drains.
- **Dermatology**: Referral may be indicated if there is skin breakdown, such as peristomal or periwound, which is unresponsive to routine care, if contact dermatitis occurs because of contact with adhesives or barrier products, and if fungal infections, such as candidiasis under a pouch, occur. Referral is often needed for ostomies, fistulae, and percutaneous tubes and drains when skin breakdown occurs.

Handoff/Transition of Patients with Ostomies

Hand-off/transition procedures for patients with ostomies whether to another unit, another level of care, or to the home environment should be documented and adequate time allowed for communication, including questions from the receiving party. Information that must be covered may vary somewhat depending on the type of ostomy but generally includes:

- Demographic information, such as name, diagnoses, address, telephone number.
- List of current medications and treatments.
- Physical or cognitive impairments that may impact ability to manage the ostomy, such as vision impairment, impaired mobility, and dementia.
- The type of ostomy, including the site and any complications (discoloration, retraction, herniation, prolapse, stenosis, bleeding, laceration).
- History of ostomy (length of time in place, history of complications, etc.)
- Current size, condition, and appearance of stoma.
- Type of ostomy supplies and equipment needed.
- Review of education provided to the patient/family.
- Contact information for ostomy specialist.
- Dietary guidelines, including foods to avoid.
- Activity level and restrictions (such as limited lifting, avoiding strenuous exercise).
- Follow-up appointments.

Practice Test

1. A 57-year-old male is diagnosed with stage III cancer of the bladder with invasion of the muscle tissue. Which primary treatment is *MOST* common?

a. partial or segmental cystectomy
b. interstitial radiation only
c. radical cystectomy with urinary diversion and chemotherapy
d. chemotherapy only

2. Which of the following stomal complications indicates a need for surgical intervention?

a. slight bleeding when changing stomal appliance
b. slow oozing at one area of the mucocutaneous juncture
c. slow bleeding at mucocutaneous juncture and caput medusa
d. frank bleeding from the mucocutaneous juncture

3. Within what period of time postoperatively should an ileostomy begin to excrete stool?

a. immediately
b. 24 to 48 hours
c. 2 to 3 days
d. 4 to 5 days

4. A male patient develops painful red pustular lesions about the peristomal area. The most likely diagnosis is

a. candidiasis.
b. folliculitis.
c. contact dermatitis.
d. trauma.

5. A patient with a colostomy develops herpes zoster with lesions in the peristomal area. The draining lesions are interfering with pouch adhesion. The *BEST* solution is to

a. apply hydrocolloid dressing to lesions.
b. apply barrier paste to lesions.
c. leave appliance off until the lesions heal.
d. mechanically debride lesions by washing and drying.

6. Which is the most effective type of pouching system for a retracted stoma?

a. concave pouching system
b. large pouching system without rigid rings
c. transparent pouching system
d. convex pouching system with a belt

7. In the PLISSIT model for communicating about sexuality, at which level should the nurse discuss topics such as the use of lubricants and pouch covers?

a. level one
b. level two
c. level three
d. level four

8. Peristomal abscess is most commonly associated with

a. Crohn's disease.
b. systemic bacterial infection.
c. paralytic ileus.
d. ulcerative colitis.

9. Which is the *MOST* common method to ensure correct placement of the stoma during surgery?

a. careful written instructions
b. marking site with permanent marker or tattoo
c. marking site by making circular scratches with a small-gauge needle
d. photograph of abdomen with site indicated

10. Which type of colostomy creates one or two stomas, usually in the upper abdomen in the middle or on the right side?

a. descending
b. transverse
c. ascending
d. end

11. A loop colostomy is usually performed for

a. simplicity of procedure.
b. inflammatory bowel disease.
c. permanent fecal diversion.
d. short-term fecal diversion.

12. When a patient is doing a colostomy irrigation, what is the correct level for the bottom of the irrigation bag?

a. above the head
b. shoulder level
c. level with the stoma
d. level with the umbilicus

13. Which of the following groups of symptoms indicates obstruction of an ileostomy?

a. dry mouth and tongue, poor skin turgor, weight loss, diarrhea, and lethargy
b. high fever, abdominal cramping, dry mouth, poor skin turgor, and bloody diarrhea
c. palpitations, lethargy, fatigue, tinnitus, dyspnea, and headache
d. edematous stoma, high-pitched bowel sounds, obvious peristaltic waves, distension, dry mouth, abdominal pain, nausea, and vomiting

14. Which of the following is most important to avoid fluid and electrolyte imbalance with an ileostomy?

a. increase intake of high fiber foods to slow absorption
b. increase intake of water with diarrhea
c. take routine antidiarrheal medication
d. monitor intake and output

15. What is the correct volume and type of fluid to use for an ileostomy lavage?

a. 500 to 1500 mL warm tap water
b. 500 mL normal saline
c. 100 mL warm tap water
d. 30 to 50 mL normal saline

16. After ileostomy takedown, the BEST functional result is

a. 8 to10 stools per day with no incontinence.
b. 6 to 8 stools per day with nighttime incontinence.
c. 4 to 5 stools per day with no or little incontinence.
d. 6 to 8 stools per day with occasional day and night incontinence.

17. A patient with a loop ileostomy and a retained distal segment of bowel has copious anal discharge of mucus. The most likely cause is

a. normal mucus production.
b. diversion colitis.
c. anastomotic leak.
d. fluid and electrolyte imbalance.

18. In which instance is the surgical intervention of a strictureplasty appropriate for treating Crohn's disease?

a. when the stricture created by the disease is excessively long or several diseased portions of the bowel connect to one another
b. when a diseased portion of the bowel connects to a healthy portion of the bowel
c. when both the colon and the rectum are infected by the disease
d. surgical interventions are contraindicated in the case of Crohn's disease

19. Which of the following complies with the AMA guidelines for informed consent for a patient facing surgery for severe inflammatory bowel disease?

a. the patient is advised to have the ileostomy with Kock pouch because the surgeon has more experience with that procedure
b. the patient is provided a brief summary of possible complications
c. the patient is provided with a number of surgical options
d. the patient is advised to relax and focus on thinking positively

20. Megacolon is associated with which of the following disorders?

a. necrotizing enterocolitis
b. Hirschsprung's disease
c. ulcerative colitis
d. Crohn's disease

21. An imperforate anus with no external opening but rectum in normal position with normal function and no connection to the GU tract is classified as

a. atypical anomalies.
b. low anomalies.
c. intermediate anomalies.
d. high anomalies.

22. Which of the following symptoms are typical of an overactive neurogenic bladder?

a. dribbling
b. straining to urinate
c. urgency
d. retention

23. If the peristomal skin about an ileostomy becomes irritated, which medication(s) may be indicated?

a. oral antibiotics
b. topical corticosteroid spray
c. topical corticosteroid spray and nystatin powder
d. topical antibiotic ointment

24. What change in ileostomy care is common during pregnancy?

a. no changes
b. change in size of appliances
c. diet modifications
d. decrease in ileostomy activity

25. The most common colorectal cancers are

a. adenocarcinomas.
b. lymphomas.
c. melanomas.
d. sarcomas.

26. The nurse is teaching a 45-year-old woman with a colostomy to do irrigations. The nurse has prepared written directions and a video, but the patient ignores them, picks up the equipment, and looks at each part, trying to figure it out. The patient's learning style is probably

a. auditory.
b. visual.
c. kinesthetic.
d. mixed.

27. A 30-year-old woman is hospitalized with severe depression and is incontinent of urine, although the urinary system is normal. The most appropriate nursing diagnosis is

a. functional urinary incontinence.
b. stress urinary incontinence.
c. overflow urinary incontinence.
d. urge urinary incontinence.

28. Which foods should be included in the diet of those with an ileostomy to reduce odor?

a. spinach and parsley
b. milk products
c. fish
d. broccoli and asparagus

29. Which agents can be used by those with ileostomies to treat constipation?

a. osmotic agents, such as Milk of Magnesia®
b. stimulant agents (such as Dulcolax®)
c. mineral oil
d. stool softeners, such as Colace®

30. A 72-year-old female is being discharged from the acute hospital with a colostomy. She is intelligent and cooperative, but is very nervous about caring for her colostomy at home, despite demonstrations and practice. Which is the MOST effective solution?

a. a home health agency referral
b. printed materials about colostomy care
c. a video showing colostomy care
d. instruction of family member to assist

31. Ureteral stents are placed postoperatively with a urostomy. On day three, the urine becomes cloudy with purulent discharge. Which action is indicated?

a. stent removal
b. gentle irrigation with 5 to 10 mL of normal saline
c. irrigation under pressure with 5 to 10 mL of normal saline
d. surgical revision

32. One of the *FIRST* indications of urostomy infection is

a. change in character and/or amount of urine.
b. fever and chills.
c. backache.
d. nausea and vomiting.

33. The *BEST* method to obtain a urine specimen for a culture and sensitivity from a patient with a urostomy is to

a. drain urine from the urostomy bag into a sterile container.
b. remove bag, cleanse peristomal skin, and hold sterile container below stoma.
c. remove bag, apply a new bag, and drain urine from the new bag into a sterile container.
d. remove bag, cleanse peristomal skin, and catheterize stoma with #14 straight catheter to obtain specimen.

34. Which is the *BEST* method to manage mucus in the urine after a urostomy?

a. increase fluid intake
b. acidify urine
c. irrigate urostomy
d. limit dairy products

35. Which of the following medications may not be absorbed completely or at all with continent cutaneous fecal diversions?

a. liquid medications
b. enteric-coated medications
c. uncoated medications
d. parenteral medications

36. Which of the following sets of symptoms would most likely indicate pouchitis for an individual with fecal diversion?

a. decrease in frequency of stools, abdominal pain, itching, and fever
b. increase in frequency of stools, dehydration, abdominal pain, and fever
c. itching, dehydration, bloody stools, and fever.
d. decrease in frequency of stools, dehydration, and fever

37. Which is the *MOST* appropriate method of cleansing the perianal area after ileal pouch anal anastomosis (IPAA)?

a. scrub the area with soap and water
b. rinse with warm water using a squirt bottle or spray
c. wash the area gently with povidone-iodine solution
d. wash gently with chlorhexidine gluconate 4% (Hibiclens®) solution

38. Which of the following breakfast choices is best to maintain acidic urine after continent cutaneous urinary diversions?

a. fruit plate, yogurt, and tea
b. orange juice, sliced bananas with yogurt, milk
c. cheese, sliced oranges and apples, and milk
d. cranberry juice, scrambled eggs, whole grain toast, and prunes

39. What is the target intubation schedule for one month after surgery for continent cutaneous urinary diversion?

a. every 2 hours during the day and every 3 hours at night
b. every 3 hours during the day and every 4 hours at night
c. every 4 hours during the day and every 5 hours at night
d. every 5 hours during the day and every 6 hours at night

40. Which of the following is utilized to promote bladder control after removal of the postoperative Foley catheter for orthotopic neobladder?

a. pelvic floor/Kegel exercises
b. scheduled straight catheterizations
c. scheduled urination every 2 to 4 hours indefinitely
d. fluid restriction in the evening

41. Where do most anorectal fistulae originate?

a. perineal skin
b. rectum
c. anal glands
d. anal sphincter

42. What type of nutritional support is indicated with enterocutaneous fistulae affecting both the small intestine and the colon?

a. enteral nutrition
b. total parenteral nutrition (TPN)
c. oral liquid diet
d. oral soft diet

43. A fistula that drains 300 mL in 24 hours would be classified by volume as

a. low output.
b. small to medium output.
c. high output.
d. extreme output.

44. Using the Parks classification system for anorectal fistulae, how would a fistula that extends from the internal sphincter, down to the perineum, and up to a blind tract or into the rectum be classified?

a. intersphincteric
b. transsphincteric
c. suprasphincteric
d. extrasphincteric

45. Which treatment option should be used *FIRST* for peristomal hyperplasia about an enteral feeding tube?

a. cauterization with silver nitrate
b. application of topical corticosteroid (such as triamcinolone or Kenalog)
c. debridement
d. resiting of tube

46. The *FIRST* step in cauterization of peristomal hyperplasia with silver nitrate sticks is to

a. moisten the silver nitrate sticks with sterile water.
b. reapply 2 to 3 times weekly until resolved.
c. run the tip of the silver nitrate stick over the hyperplastic tissue using a rolling motion.
d. apply a skin barrier around the hyperplastic tissue.

47. How much space should be left between the external bumper and the skin to prevent excessive traction and buried bumper syndrome?

a. 0.5 cm
b. 1.0 cm
c. 1.5 cm
d. 2 cm

48. Which of the following is indicated to prevent occlusion of enteral feeding tubes used for intermittent or continuous feeding?

a. flush with 30 mL water every 8 hours or after feedings and medication administration
b. flush with 30 mL water every 8 hours and before feedings and medication administration
c. flush with 30 mL of water every 4 hours
d. flush with 30 mL of water every 4 hours and before and after feedings and medication administration

49. The patient has a percutaneous endoscopic gastrostomy (PEG) and has developed leakage about the tube. What INITIAL intervention is indicated?

a. check the balloon to ensure adequate inflation
b. stabilize the tube with the bumper and external stabilizer
c. replace the tube
d. apply barrier ointment

50. Which is the BEST method for nighttime management of a urostomy?

a. empty the bag right before bed
b. attach a leg bag to the appliance to hold overflow
c. limit fluid intake in the evening to decrease urinary output
d. attach a long tube and an overnight urinary drainage bag

51. A patient with an ileostomy has developed hyponatremia when the sodium value drops to

a. <145 mEq.
b. <135 mEq.
c. <130 mEq.
d. <125 mEq.

52. A low profile percutaneous feeding tube is recommended for pediatric patients because

a. it is less uncomfortable.
b. it is easier to insert.
c. it is less likely to become dislodged.
d. it has fewer complications.

53. Which of the following is a critical element of active listening?

a. providing feedback
b. remaining passive
c. focusing only the speaker's words
d. making constant eye contact

54. Which of the following is a measure to prevent buried bumper syndrome with a percutaneous endoscopic gastrostomy (PEG) tube?

a. rotate the tube daily
b. place a dressing under the external fixation device
c. flush the tube before feedings
d. mark the tube where it exits the skin

55. When using a closed suction system to manage a high-output fistula, the suction catheter is positioned

a. 4 to 5 cm inside the fistula orifice.
b. 1 to 2 cm inside the fistula orifice.
c. 4 cm away from the fistula orifice.
d. next to the fistula orifice.

56. How long after a percutaneous endoscopic gastrostomy (PEG) is performed is the tract usually mature and well-healed enough for placement of a balloon gastrostomy tube (G-tube)?

a. 4 to 7 days
b. 2 to 4 weeks
c. 1 to 2 months
d. 3 to 4 months

57. If a patient complains of difficulty keeping a seal of an ostomy appliance because of a bulge on one side of the stoma, the most likely cause is

a. parastomal hernia.
b. tumor.
c. abscess.
d. constipation.

58. Management of severe stomal stenosis usually requires

a. intermittent use of a dilator.
b. surgical repair.
c. regular use of a dilator.
d. dietary modifications.

59. If a patient with a colostomy has a new onset of loose stools, the nurse should initially review the patient's

a. medication history.
b. activity level.
c. fluid intake.
d. food history.

60. If an ostomy pouch has a drainable spout, it is usually positioned at

a. 12 o'clock.
b. 9 o'clock.
c. 6 o'clock.
d. 3 o'clock.

61. An ostomy pouch with a deodorizing gas filter works best with

a. any type of output.
b. formed stool.
c. semi-liquid stool.
d. liquid stool.

62. When preparing a cut-to-fit ostomy pouch, the patient should be taught to

a. trace the stoma on a piece of plastic wrap.
b. measure the stoma diameter with a ruler.
c. start with a small opening and gradually enlarge.
d. make a template out of a piece of paper and use as a pattern.

63. Stomal retraction is most common in patients who are

a. young adults.
b. older adults.
c. very thin.
d. obese.

64. A clear pouch should be used over the stoma in the immediate postoperative period in order to

a. monitor output.
b. begin patient acceptance of stoma.
c. allow stomal assessment.
d. prevent mechanical trauma.

65. If the patient is markedly obese with a very large abdomen, the stoma

a. should be sited as usual.
b. may need to be sited higher than usual.
c. may need to be sited lower than usual.
d. should be on the usual beltline.

66. If, following an emergent traumatic injury, a 25-year old patient required a colectomy and permanent end colostomy, but the patient has become increasingly withdrawn and shows evidence of suicidal ideation, the most appropriate response is to

a. refer the patient for psychological counseling.
b. ask a volunteer ostomate to visit the patient.
c. suggest the patient join a support group.
d. encourage the patient to participate in care.

67. If a patient develops granulomas at the peristomal skin/stoma juncture, the treatment of choice is usually

a. surgical debridement.
b. mechanical debridement.
c. electrical cauterization.
d. silver nitrate cauterization.

68. Sodium phosphate bowel prep is usually more acceptable to patients than polyethylene glycol preparations because sodium phosphate

a. works faster.
b. spares electrolytes.
c. has a pleasant taste.
d. has low volume.

69. The two primary concerns of ostomy patients are

a. inconvenience and discomfort.
b. embarrassment and shame.
c. odor control and leakage.
d. pain and physical limitations.

70. When assessing the postoperative condition of a fecal stoma, the nurse expects the stoma to be

a. flush with the skin.
b. deep red in color.
c. light pink in color.
d. grossly edematous.

71. Ideally a stoma, such as for an end ileostomy, should protrude from the skin by approximately

a. 1 to 2 cm.
b. 2 to 3 cm.
c. 3 to 4 cm.
d. 4 to 5 cm.

72. The ideal site for a stoma is in which muscle?

a. internal oblique
b. external oblique
c. rectus abdominus
d. latissimus dorsi

73. Following construction of an Indiana pouch, irrigation is usually carried out with

a. 20 to 30 mL NS two times daily.
b. 20 to 30 mL NS four times daily.
c. 30 to 60 mL NS two times daily.
d. 30 to 60 mL NS four times daily.

74. The continent ileostomy (Kock pouch) is currently

a. the procedure of choice for ulcerative colitis.
b. used primarily as a backup for IPAA failure.
c. no longer advised because of complications.
d. used only for patients with Crohn's disease.

75. The ileal pouch anal anastomosis (IPAA) is not routinely recommended for patients with Crohn's disease because of

a. increased risk of pouch failure/pouch-associated fistulae.
b. increased risk of postoperative hemorrhage.
c. patient resistance to the procedure.
d. prolonged period of healing and limited mobility required.

76. Patients with a perineal wound should be reminded to avoid using a donut cushion because

a. it provides no relief from discomfort.
b. it causes increased blood flow and risk of bleeding.
c. it causes pulling of the incision and decreased blood flow.
d. it increases the risk of skin irritation.

77. If a patient with inflammatory bowel disease presents with hair loss, weight loss, balance problems, decreased energy and fatigue, the nurse should suspect

a. electrolyte imbalance.
b. systemic infection.
c. depression/anxiety.
d. malnutrition.

78. The most common surgical procedure for Crohn's disease is removal of the

a. terminal jejunum and proximal ileum.
b. terminal ileum and cecum.
c. cecum and proximal ascending colon.
d. ileum only.

79. With extensive ulcerative colitis, the distance (measured from the anal verge) of involved tissue is

a. 20 cm.
b. 35 to 40 cm.
c. >60 cm.
d. entire colon.

80. If a patient with an ileal pouch anal anastomosis (IPAA) experiences anal burning and loose stools after eating certain foods, the treatment may include

a. bile salt binding agents.
b. simethicone.
c. loperamide.
d. corticosteroid.

81. If a patient has developed skin irritation about a biliary tube, the best solution is to apply

a. barrier paste.
b. barrier cream.
c. barrier wafer cut to fit around tube.
d. alcohol-free liquid skin barrier.

82. The most common cause of bladder cancer is

a. genetic predisposition.
b. smoking (tobacco).
c. alcohol abuse.
d. environmental toxins.

83. If siting both a fecal and a urinary stoma, the urinary stoma should be

a. the same height as the fecal stoma.
b. at least one inch lower than the fecal stoma.
c. at least one inch higher than the fecal stoma.
d. on the opposite side of the abdomen from the fecal stoma.

84. A patient with an ileostomy should be advised that the best way to take fluids is

a. by themselves without food.
b. together with food.
c. before eating.
d. after eating.

85. What percentage of patients with an ileal pouch anal anastomosis (IPAA) develop chronic pouchitis?

a. 5%
b. 10%
c. 30%
d. 40%

86. If a patient has familial adenomatous polyposis (FAP), the chance of developing colon cancer by age 40 is

a. 100%.
b. 75%.
c. 50%.
d. 25%.

87. A moderate output enterocutaneous fistula is one with an output of

a. 100 to 200 mL/24 hours.
b. 500 to 700 mL/24 hours.
c. 200 to 500 mL/24 hours.
d. 50 to 100 mL/24 hours.

88. Modifiable risk factors for the development of colorectal cancer include

a. age.
b. high fat/low fiber diet.
c. disease.
d. genetic predisposition.

89. If the physician has ordered that a nephrostomy tube be flushed because of mucus and sediment in the urine, the irrigation should be done with

a. 30 to 40 mL NS.
b. 20 to 30 mL NS.
c. 10 to 20 mL NS.
d. 5 to 10 mL NS.

90. Which of the following is characteristic of ulcerative colitis?

a. superficial mucosal penetration
b. patchy areas of inflammation
c. presence of fistulae
d. presence of granulomas

91. The first step in managing stomal trauma is to

a. change the type/size of pouch.
b. apply topical antibiotic to prevent infection.
c. identify the cause.
d. apply skin barrier cream to the stoma.

92. If a patient has a proximal enterocutaneous fistula, the primary concern is

a. odor.
b. cutaneous periwound condition.
c. pain.
d. nutrition.

93. Most cases of metastatic melanoma to the gastrointestinal system occur in the

a. rectum.
b. stomach.
c. small intestine.
d. colon.

94. A patient with a high output ileostomy should avoid drinking excessive hypotonic fluids, such as water, fruit juice, and soda, because they

a. increase risk of hypernatremia.
b. increase risk of hyponatremia.
c. can lead to increased thirst.
d. increase risk of leakage.

95. If a patient has an ileal pouch anal anastomosis (IPAA) and has become pregnant, the patient should be advised that she may experience

a. increased frequency of stools and fecal incontinence.
b. increased incidence of pouchitis.
c. decreased frequency of stools.
d. increased risk of stillbirth.

96. If a patient is undergoing video capsule endoscopy for Crohn's disease, a primary concern is

a. infection.
b. capsule retention.
c. intestinal perforation.
d. allergic response.

97. If an 80-year-old male is too frail to carry out the irrigations independently and his 72-year-old wife is still confused about the procedure, which of the following is likely the BEST plan?

a. transfer the patient to a convalescent hospital
b. keep the patient in the hospital until the wife is more capable
c. advise the patient to hire someone to assist with the irrigations
d. refer the patient to a home health agency for assistance

98. If, when the urostomy appliance is removed after 4 days, the skin is clear but there is erosion in the peristomal area of the barrier of the appliance, this means that

a. the appliance should be changed less frequently.
b. the appliance could be changed more frequently.
c. the appliance performed as expected.
d. the appliance was the wrong size.

99. If a 64-year-old female client has recently had surgery for colon cancer and has a colostomy, but the client has been resistive to educational efforts and refuses to look at the colostomy, the MOST appropriate intervention is

a. remain supportive and encourage client to express feelings.
b. remind the client that she will have to soon assume self-care.
c. insist that the client assist in care of the colostomy.
d. ask a family member to assume responsibility for colostomy care.

100. If a Vietnamese immigrant patient had surgery for a bowel resection and colostomy but has not requested pain medicine in the 6 hours after returning from the recovery room to his room on the surgical unit, the nurse should assume the patient

a. has no pain.
b. is insensitive to pain.
c. is reluctant to complain of pain.
d. has not recovered from anesthesia.

101. When teaching a patient to irrigate a colostomy, how much fluid should the patient be advised to use for the irrigation?

a. 200 to 500 mL
b. 500 to 700 mL
c. 500 to 1000 mL
d. 1000 to 1500 mL

102. Which of the following is the best choice to protect the skin from drainage from a high-output fistula?

a. moisture barrier powder
b. skin barrier spray
c. absorbant dressings
d. moisture barrier cream

103. When siting the stoma for a woman who is 6 months pregnant, the stoma site should be

a. in the same position as for non-pregnant patients.
b. in the same horizontal plane as the umbilicus.
c. more medial than the usual site.
d. more lateral than the usual site.

104. Most bacteria that is ingested orally is eliminated by

a. gastric alkalinity.
b. gastric acidity.
c. intestinal bile.
d. intestinal villi.

105. Absorption of nutrients, electrolytes, vitamins, and minerals takes place primarily in the

a. stomach.
b. small intestine.
c. ascending colon.
d. descending colon.

106. Penrose drains are usually kept in a wound postoperatively for

a. 1 to 2 days.
b. 2 to 3 days.
c. 3 to 5 days.
d. 6 to 7 days.

107. Most colorectal lymphomas are located in the

a. cecum/ascending colon.
b. transverse colon.
c. descending colon
d. sigmoid colon/rectum.

108. If a patient is diagnosed with rectal cancer, which of the following TNM classifications generally indicate the need for transanal excision only?

a. T4
b. T3N2
c. T2N0
d. T1N0

109. Most electrolyte loss occurs through

a. urine.
b. respirations.
c. feces.
d. perspiration.

110. If a colonoscopy shows a fragmented polyp with invasive cancer, the likely treatment will be

a. remove the polyp and observe the patient.
b. adjuvant therapy only.
c. colectomy, removal of lymph nodes, and possible diversion.
d. colectomy, removal of lymph nodes, diversion, and adjuvant therapy.

111. Carcinoid tumors are most common in which of the following ethnic groups?

a. Asians
b. African Americans
c. Hispanics
d. Caucasians

112. Which of the following makes patients with Crohn's disease more refractory to treatment?

a. older age
b. obesity
c. alcohol use
d. smoking

113. A patient with Crohn's disease is especially at risk for which of the following vitamin deficiencies?

a. B12
b. B6
c. C
d. D

114. With ulcerative colitis, which of the following is an indication for urgent surgery?

a. chronic steroid dependency
b. refractory disease
c. adenocarcinoma
d. toxic megacolon

115. If a patient has a subtotal colectomy with ileostomy and a Hartman's pouch for Crohn's disease, the patient should be told to expect

a. no issues with the Hartman's pouch.
b. to feel the urge to defecate and pass mucus periodically.
c. to feel no urge to defecate but leak mucus.
d. periodic cramping pain in the Hartman's pouch.

116. If a male patient who is 6 weeks postoperative with an ileal pouch anal anastomosis (IPAA) complains of difficulty achieving an erection and engaging in sexual activity and seems quite distressed, the MOST appropriate referral is to a

a. urologist.
b. gastroenterologist.
c. sex therapist.
d. psychologist.

117. If a patient with Crohn's disease is considering surgery to create an ileostomy, the most important role of the nurse is to

a. provide encouragement and reassurance.
b. stress the positive aspects of an ileostomy.
c. stress the negative aspects of an ileostomy.
d. provide information about the procedure.

118. When a patient undergoing a 3-stage proctocolectomy and ileal pouch anal anastomosis (IPAA) procedure has the end ileostomy changed to a temporary loop ileostomy, the patient is especially at increased risk of

a. infection.
b. dehydration.
c. dehiscence.
d. hemorrhage.

119. If a patient has an ileostomy, which type of foods is most indicated to thicken the stool?

a. fats
b. dairy foods
c. starchy foods
d. high protein foods

120. Which of the following is a contraindication to negative pressure wound therapy (NPWT) for an enterocutaneous fistula?

a. exposed bowel at wound base
b. lack of pseudostoma
c. no potential for spontaneous closure
d. indications of infection in the wound

Answer Key and Explanations

1. C: The most standard treatment for cancer that has invaded the muscle is radical cystectomy with urinary diversion. Chemotherapy may be done prior to or after surgery to improve survival rates, because recurrence rates are about 50%. In males, the bladder, prostate, seminal vesicles, and perivesical tissues are removed; in females, the bladder, uterus, ovaries, fallopian tubes, urethra, and anterior vaginal wall are removed. Urinary diversions may include an ileal conduit or an internal pouch, such as the Indiana pouch or neobladder (formed from part of the intestine).

2. D: Frank bleeding from the mucocutaneous juncture may indicate bleeding from a mesenteric artery, requiring surgery to open the incision and ligate the artery. A slight bleeding when changing of stomal appliance relates to mechanical trauma to the mucosa and is normal, unless it continues. Slow oozing usually stops, but may require cauterization. Oozing of blood may be caused by antiplatelet drugs, such as salicylates. Slow bleeding along with caput medusa (distention of veins about the umbilicus) is a complication related to portal hypertension.

3. B: An ileostomy should begin to function and excrete stool by 24 to 48 hours postoperatively, because digested food passes quickly into the small intestine in liquid form. A colostomy, however, may not pass stool for 4 to 5 days, varying somewhat with the position of the colostomy, which affects reabsorption of liquids. Because kidneys constantly produce urine, an ureterostomy should immediately produce urine. Stomas should be observed carefully to ensure that they are functioning properly. Delayed function may indicate obstruction or other complications.

4. B: Folliculitis is inflammation of the hair follicles by staphylococcus aureus. The lesions are often pustular, red, and painful. Folliculitis usually results from slight nicks in the skin from shaving with a razor, from friction, or from occlusion. Candidiasis is a fungal infection that causes inflammation with burning and itching and red patches, related to prolonged moisture on skin, usually from secretions or leakage under the pouch. Contact dermatitis may result from a hypersensitivity reaction to a particular chemical or product in the pouching system. Skin may be red, draining, and painful. Chemical trauma from secretions may look similar: red, draining, and painful.

5. A: Hydrocolloid dressing may be used to prevent fluid from herpetic lesions from interfering with the pouching system. Herpes zoster and herpes simplex, both viral illnesses, remain dormant, but can be triggered by illness or stress and can erupt in the peristomal area. Antiviral treatments may be used to speed healing. Herpetic lesions in the peristomal area may be irritated by pouch adhesive. While cool moist compresses may provide some relief from discomfort, the lesions should be allowed to open and dry on their own (usually within 2 to 3 weeks).

6. D: A convex pouching system with a belt is used for a retracted stoma because it fits snugly about the stoma to prevent leakage. Retraction occurs when the stoma pulls below the skin level. This is caused by tension below the stoma, which can be from a variety of factors, including excessive scar formation, obesity, inadequate stoma length, recurrence of active Crohn's disease, and improper excision of skin. In severe cases, achieving a seal about the stoma may be very difficult, and may require surgical revision.

7. C: Specific suggestions are given at Level 3 in the PLISSIT model:

- Level 1—Permission: giving the person permission to have feelings or attitudes and to do or not do something.
- Level 2—Limited Information: providing factual information, specifically related to needs and concerns of patient, that helps dispel misconceptions and fears.
- Level 3—Specific Suggestions: making recommendations when a person needs to take action or seek treatment with medical guidance.
- Level 4—Intensive Therapy: referring the patient to an appropriate specialist, for example if reconstructive surgery or psychotherapy is needed.

8. A: Peristomal abscess is common with active Crohn's disease distal to the stoma. Crohn's disease is a form of inflammatory bowel disease in which ulcerations occur in the small and sometimes in the large intestines. Peristomal abscess is characterized by open (from fistulae) and closed lesions that are painful, swollen, and erythematous. Peristomal abscess may also occur after stomal revision, because of contamination from skin bacteria. Colostomy irrigation may result in perforation that causes abscess formation. A peristomal abscess rarely heals spontaneously but requires surgical incision and drainage.

9. B: The most common method to ensure correct placement of the stoma during surgery is to mark the site with a permanent marker. The site is marked with an X or circle, and is usually covered with a transparent dressing to protect the markings. Markings will usually last for 1 to 3 weeks, but patients should be provided a marking pen and additional dressings in case markings fade. Tattooing is the most permanent method of marking, but is painful for the patient. Making circular scratches in the epidermis with a small-gauge needle is not recommended, because the break in the skin can lead to infection.

10. B: A transverse colostomy creates one or two stomas in the transverse colon, usually in the upper abdomen, in the middle or on the right side. A descending (sigmoid) colostomy (most common) creates a stoma from the end of the sigmoid colon, usually in the lower left abdomen. An ascending colostomy creates a stoma from the ascending portion of the colon on the right side of the abdomen. An end colostomy is a temporary procedure or a permanent procedure where a stoma is created proximal to an inoperable carcinoma to allow for fecal diversion and to prolong life.

11. D: A loop colostomy is usually performed for short-term fecal diversion. A loop colostomy creates one stoma with two openings, one for stool and the other for mucus, usually in the transverse colon. A supporting rod may be in place to maintain the stoma's position. This procedure is relatively easy and can be reversed in a simple operation. Indications include trauma, conditions requiring the bowel to heal and rest, such as cancer, and (in children) major pelvic surgery.

12. B: The bag should be at shoulder level. Follow this procedure:

1. Hang the bag with 500 to 1500 mL lukewarm water, with the bottom at shoulder level, and release air bubbles from the tubing.
2. Sit on or near toilet. Apply a long irrigation sleeve, placing the end into the toilet.
3. Lubricate the cone nozzle and insert it about 3 inches into stoma in the direction of the colon.
4. Holding the cone firmly in place to retain the fluid, open the clamp and let the fluid flow into colon slowly, over about 5 to 10 minutes. Hold the cone in place for a few seconds and then remove it.

5. Drain fecal output into the toilet for 10 to 15 minutes. The initial flow of fluids is usually followed by fecal material within 15 minutes.
6. Dry and clamp the end of the irrigation sleeve. Keep the bag in place for up to an hour if stool continues to drain. Remove the irrigation sleeve, cleanse peristomal area, and apply the pouch.

13. D: Indications of ileostomy obstruction include edematous stoma, high-pitched bowel sounds, obvious peristaltic waves, distension, dry mouth, abdominal pain, nausea, and vomiting. Obstruction is usually related to high-fiber foods. Other complications include

- Fluid and electrolyte imbalance: mouth and tongue dry, skin turgor poor, weight loss, diarrhea, and lethargy.
- Vitamin B12 deficiency: palpitations, lethargy, fatigue, tinnitus, dyspnea, and headache.
- Pouchitis: high fever, abdominal cramping, dry mouth, poor skin turgor, and bloody diarrhea.

14. D: Monitoring intake and output is most important in preventing fluid and electrolyte imbalance, along with ensuring adequate nutrition. During episodes of diarrhea, the patient should substitute water with Gatorade® or a similar sports drink designed to replenish electrolytes and supply nutrition. With electrolyte imbalance, increasing the oral intake of fluids is not sufficient, because these fluids will be excreted through the kidneys and may not correct the electrolyte imbalance. If stools are too liquid, the patient can increase fiber and, if stools are too dry, increase sodium. Antidiarrheal agents should be taken only as necessary when dietary changes are not sufficient, never routinely.

15. D: Lavage is NOT the same as an irrigation, which uses large volumes of fluid. About 30 to 50 mL of normal saline (NS) is used to prevent further dehydration, instilled with a catheter-tipped piston or bulb syringe with a 14 to 16 Fr catheter attached. Lavage is usually done after an abdominal x-ray has determined that food is the cause of a blockage.

1. Apply irrigation sleeve with the end in the toilet.
2. Do a digital exam to determine the direction of intestine.
3. Lubricate the catheter and gently insert it approximately 12 to 15 cms.
4. Slowly inject normal saline into the intestine and then slowly aspirate the entire amount with light to moderate pressure.
5. Repeat the procedure until the blockage is relieved.

16. C: After ileostomy takedown, the best functional result is 4 to 5 stools per day with no incontinence, but most procedures result in (at best) 95% continence during the daytime and 90% continence during the night. The ileoanal reservoir is usually quite small after surgery, so 8 to 10 stools per day is not unusual in the immediate postoperative period, putting the person at risk for fluid and electrolyte imbalances; the reservoir capacity will expand and stool frequency should decrease over a 6 to 12-month period.

17. B: While some anal mucus discharge is normal, copious discharge is often associated with diversion colitis, in which the distal segment becomes inflamed. Treatment includes rectal irrigation and topical steroids, as well as oral antibiotics. The perianal area should be cleansed and protective cream or ointment applied to prevent irritation of the skin. The mucus fistula should be checked each time the appliance is changed and discharged mucus gently wiped from the opening. The stoma should remain pink. Changes in color or swelling may indicate compromised circulation or infection.

18. B: A strictureplasty is a surgical procedure that widens the narrowed bowel in cases of chronic inflammation or scar tissue, such as that occurring with Crohn's disease. In this procedure, no aspect of the intestine is removed, preserving the bowel length. A strictureplasty is indicated when a diseased portion of the bowel connects to a healthy portion. The procedure widens the narrowed or scarred portion, and maintains the intestinal flow. If the strictures are extensive, part of the intestine will require removal (resection). If both the colon and the rectum are infected by the disease, the entire colon may need to be removed (colectomy). Approximately 70-90% of patients affected by Crohn's disease will require surgical intervention during their lifetime.

19. C: Providing the patient with a list of surgical options complies with the AMA guidelines for informed consent. Options should not be limited by a specific surgeon's area of expertise or experience, as a patient can be referred to other surgeons. The patient must be provided a complete list and explanation of possible complications, not a brief summary. While relaxing and focusing on thinking positively may have benefits, this advice is not part of informed consent.

20. B: Megacolon is associated with Hirschsprung's disease, a congenital disorder in which infants are born without intestinal ganglion nerve cells in part of or the entire colon, causing mechanical obstruction. Normally, nerves signal the colon to contract, pushing the stool through the colon, but the absence of propulsion in the segments without ganglions causes the fecal material to accumulate. Affected areas almost always include the rectum and distal colon, but in rare instances can "skip" segments and involve the entire colon and the small intestine. As fecal material collects, the segment of the bowel proximal to the defect distends, creating megacolon.

21. B: Imperforate anus with low anomalies: no external opening, but the rectum is otherwise in normal position through the puborectalis muscle, with normal function and no connection to the genitourinary tract.

22. C: An overactive neurogenic bladder is characterized by urgency, frequency, dysuria, urinary tract infection, and fever, while an underactive neurogenic bladder results in incontinence, dribbling, straining, inability to urinate, and retention. Neurogenic bladder is bladder dysfunction from lesions of the peripheral or central nervous system with traumatic or congenital etiologies or resulting from cerebrovascular accident or diabetic neuropathy. Nerve damage can cause an underactive bladder, which is unable to contract effectively to empty the bladder, or an overactive bladder, which contracts frequently and ineffectually.

23. C: Peristomal irritation, usually caused by chemical trauma from secretions, may be treated with corticosteroid (Kenalog®) spray, to reduce inflammation, and nystatin (Mycostatin®) powder, for fungal infections, which are common under appliances. Oral antibiotics are not indicated unless there are signs of folliculitis (pustules, erythema, and warmth). Topical antibiotics are not indicated for irritation, and ointments should not be used under appliances, as they will prevent the appliance from adhering. Alternative methods include applying a Stomahesive® wafer directly over irritated skin or applying karaya powder and then a karaya gum washer.

24. B: As the abdomen enlarges, the stoma often also enlarges and changes shape, becoming more oval. The stoma should be measured from time to time, and appliance size changed as necessary. The stoma usually returns to normal shortly after delivery. An ileostomy may be more active during pregnancy because of increased pressure. While adequate fluid intake and nutrition are important, no special diet modifications are indicated. There is a slight chance of blockage as the fetus grows and applies pressure, causing distention and pain. Treatment includes liquid diet and rest or intravenous fluids to rest the intestines.

25. A: Adenocarcinomas develop from epithelial tissue in adenomatous polyps and account for 90 to 95% of all colorectal cancers. Lymphomas are rare primary tumors that occur primarily in the rectum, while secondary metastatic tumors occur primarily in the colon. Melanomas are rare tumors that usually metastasize from other parts of body, accounting for <2% of colorectal cancers. Sarcomas (leiomyosarcoma) develop from smooth muscle and account for <2% of colorectal cancers, but >50% metastasize. Carcinoids are slow-growing tumors that rarely spread, most commonly found in the rectum and accounting for <1% of colorectal cancers.

26. C: Kinesthetic learners learn best by handling, doing, and practicing and should be allowed to handle supplies and equipment with minimal instruction. They benefit from demonstrating their understanding by doing the procedure. Visual learners learn best by seeing and reading, and they benefit from written directions, videos, diagrams, pictures, and demonstrations. Auditory learners learn best by listening and talking, so procedures should be explained during demonstrations. Auditory learners benefit from audiotapes and extra time for questions. While learning styles do vary some from person to person, all people do need learn from visual information, auditory information, and by hands-on learning. Different materials lend themselves to a different format, but where possible, the best practice when presenting information to others is to use a mixture of formats, including hands-on materials, visual, and auditory information to keep the materials engaging to all learners.

27. A: Functional urinary incontinence can occur when physical (impaired mobility) or mental (confusion, depression) disabilities prevent the person from controlling urination. Stress incontinence is characterized by small amounts of involuntary urinary leakage, often during physical activity. Overflow incontinence is characterized by small leakage of urine resulting from pressure on an over-distended bladder. Urge incontinence is caused by moderate to large amounts of involuntary urinary leakage caused by sudden urge to urinate and inability to hold urine.

28. A: Spinach and parsley have properties that help to eliminate odor in the intestinal tract. Most appliances are now odor proof, but leaking or improper cleaning of the appliance may lead to odor. If odor persists, bismuth subcarbonate tablets taken 3 to 4 times daily may effectively reduce odor. Additionally, a number of different deodorant tablets and drops are available to place inside of a pouch to reduce odor. Milk products, fish, broccoli, and asparagus may increase odor.

29. D: Stool softeners (DSS, Colace®) increase retention of fluid in the stool, helping to prevent constipation and impaction. Fiber and bulking agents may also be used. These include preparations made with methylcellulose (Citrucel®), psyllium (Metamucil®), and bran, which dissolve or swell in the intestines, promoting peristalsis. Osmotic (Milk of Magnesia®) and stimulant laxatives (Dulcolax®) should be avoided by those with ileostomies, as they can lead to increased diarrhea and electrolyte imbalance. They should be rarely used with any type of fecal diversion. Overuse can lead to bowel dysfunction. Mineral oil should not be used as a laxative.

30. A: The most effective solution is a home health agency referral, so a nurse can visit the patient in her home and provide further education and supervision. Printed materials and video are also helpful, but many people need hands-on experience and one-on-one instruction to feel secure about ostomy care. Patients are often overwhelmed with new information while in the hospital and are not able to fully comprehend what they need to do, even if they are alert and intelligent. Many people are reluctant to be assisted by family members, and they may be less motivated to be independent in care if they can depend on someone else.

31. A: In the case of suspected or confirmed infection indicated by pain, purulent discharge, or fever, the stent must be removed. Likely, antibiotics will also be prescribed. While stents are the primary management of urinary tract disease and postoperatively with a urostomy, risk of urinary tract infection is increased when any foreign body is introduced into the urinary tract. For this reason, the goal is to utilize ureteral stents as short as possible and to enforce infection prevention efforts to avoid this complication. Prior to stent insertion, a urine culture should be collected to determine (and treat) any pre-existing infection. Irrigation will not effectively treat an infection, nor would surgical revision.

32. A: While symptoms may vary, one of the first indications of a urostomy infection is usually a change in the character and/or amount of urine. The urine may become cloudy from mucus or purulent material. Hematuria may be present. Also, urine usually becomes concentrated and may be dark yellow, orange, or brownish in color and have a very strong or foul odor. Urinary output may decrease markedly. Other symptoms, such as fever, chills, back or flank pain (generally indicating infection has spread to the kidneys), and nausea and vomiting may also occur.

33. D: The best method to obtain a urine specimen from a urostomy is to remove the appliance, cleanse peristomal skin, and catheterize the stoma with a #14 straight catheter. A urine specimen should never be obtained from a bag that has been in use, because it is considered contaminated. If the stoma cannot be catheterized, an alternative method is to remove the appliance, cleanse the peristomal tissue, apply a new clean appliance, and obtain the specimen from the new bag. Do not hold a sterile cup below a stoma and attempt to obtain a specimen.

34. A: The best method to manage mucus in the urine after a urostomy is to increase fluid intake to 2 to 3 L daily to flush the mucus. Mucus production is normal. In the period immediately following, a marked increase in mucus in the urine may occur, but this will usually abate. Gentle irrigations will be done postsurgically to maintain patency of ureteral catheters. Acidifying the urine may help reduce crystal formation. Irrigating the urostomy is not recommended and may cause infection. Dairy products do not cause increased mucus.

35. B: Because of the loss of the colon, enteric-coated medications or time-release capsules spend less time in the intestine and may not be absorbed completely or at all. Uncoated tablets or liquid medications usually are absorbed; however, if food is passing through the ileostomy undigested, there may be decreased absorption of uncoated and liquid medications.

- Antidiabetics: Glucophage may not be absorbed properly.
- Birth control pills: These may not be completely absorbed, making them unreliable.
- Corticosteroids*:* Corticosteroids can cause sodium retention and fungal infection under the faceplate of the pouch because they suppress the immune system.
- Diuretics: May cause electrolyte imbalance.

36. B: One common indication of pouchitis is a steady increase in the frequency of stools. The patient may also develop fecal incontinence, watery, or bloody stools, and a feeling of urgency. Some may develop cramping abdominal pain. Dehydration and fever may occur with excessive loss of fluids. Pouchitis is a nonspecific inflammation of the mucosal lining of the internal (ileoanal, Kock, J, W, S) pouch created from part of the small intestine after colectomy. It usually occurs during the first 2 years after surgery and is most common among those with ulcerative colitis. Itching and a decrease in the frequency of stools do not indicate pouchitis.

37. B: With IPAA, seepage of fecal material and mucus from the anus may occur, especially at night. The combination of moisture and friction from walking or wiping the area with tissue can cause severe irritation, so the patient should rinse the perineal area with warm water using a squirt bottle or bulb syringe or gently wipe with cotton balls, Tucks®, or baby wipes. Patients should avoid washcloths, which are too rough, and soap, which may irritate because of alkalinity, and should pat dry, fan, or use a cool hair dryer. Preventive measures include skin barrier cream or ointment and positioning a soft dressing between buttocks.

38. D: Foods that produce acidic urine include grains and cereals, meats, cheese, corn, crackers, cranberries, eggs, pasta, nuts, rice, prunes, plums, fish, and poultry. The pH of the urine ranges normally from 4.6 to 8, in the acidic range, and patients should maintain acidity. Alkaline urine is more likely to become infected and develop crystals. Most meats and cereals produce acidic urine, but most fruits and vegetables produce alkaline urine. Drinking cranberry juice instead of orange juice can help to keep the urine acidic. Patients may also take daily vitamin C, with permission of physician.

39. D: The target intubation schedule for one month after surgery for continent cutaneous urinary diversion is usually every 5 hours during the day and every 6 hours during the night. Immediately after surgery, intubation is done every 2 hours, but as healing takes place, the time is extended until the pouch can hold increased amounts of urine. Patients must be cautioned to maintain a regular schedule to avoid infection and overdistention or rupture of the pouch.

40. A: Pelvic floor/Kegel exercises must be done both preoperatively and postoperatively. Because the neobladder does not expel urine, the abdominal muscles must tighten and the sphincter muscles relax. Scheduled urinations usually begin with every 2 hours during the day and 3 hours at night, extending time until reaching the target of every 4 hours during the day and once at night. Patients must sit to urinate and strain, often taking several minutes. Those who cannot completely empty the bladder may need to catheterize one or more times daily. Fluids should not be restricted.

41. C: Most anorectal fistulas originate in the anal glands, which are located between the layers of the anal sphincters and drain into the anal canal. If the glands become blocked and an abscess forms, it can begin to tunnel toward the surface of the skin. There may be only one tunnel or tract, or several. Abscesses can recur if they heal over at the surface. As purulent material collects beneath the healed surface, pressure builds, and it breaks through again. Anorectal fistulas are common in those with Crohn's disease. They can also occur with rectal cancer or following radiation therapy.

42. B: With enterocutaneous fistulae (extending from intestines to skin), nutritional support is provided with total parenteral nutrition (TPN) if both the small intestine and colon are involved, but enteral support if only the colon is involved. Fluid restriction and somatostatin help to decrease small bowel secretions. The most frequent causes are Crohn's disease, cancer, anastomotic leak, bowel obstruction, and sepsis. They may develop postoperatively or spontaneously. If excess pressure develops on an anastomosis, a fistula can develop. Fistulae seek weakness in tissues and thus may exit through wounds, incisions, drain sites, or compromised tissue.

43. B: A fistula that drains 300 mL in 24 hours would be classified as a small to medium output fistula. Classification systems help to characterize fistulae and assist in their management and treatment. Sometimes, more than one classification may be used to describe a fistula. Below are volume (drainage) classifications:

- Low-output fistulas drain <150 mL in 24 hours.
- Small to medium output fistulas drain 150 to 500 mL in 24 hours.
- High output fistulas drain >500 mL in 24 hours.

44. A: Intersphincteric. Parks classification for anorectal fistulae include:

- Intersphincteric: extending from the internal sphincter downward to the perineum, up to a high blind tract, or open into the rectum itself (70%).
- Transsphincteric: extending from the internal and external sphincters to the ischiorectal fossa to the perineum (25%).
- Suprasphincteric: crossing the internal sphincter to the external sphincter above the puborectalis muscles and then down to the ischioanal fossa and to the skin (5%).
- Extrasphincteric: extending from the perianal skin through the levator ani muscles and through the rectal wall (1%).
- Horseshoe: partially circling the anus, opening at both ends in the cutaneous tissue.

45. B: Topical corticosteroid cream may be effective in treating peristomal hyperplasia and is less invasive than other treatments. If corticosteroid cream is ineffective, the next step is usually cauterization with silver nitrate. Surgical debridement may be required in severe cases. Resiting may result in development of peristomal hyperplasia at the new site. Peristomal hyperplasia is an overgrowth of granulation tissue about the stoma. It usually results from irritation caused by latex tubes, tube migration, or moisture.

46. D: Care must be taken to use silver nitrate only on the granulation tissue, as it can cause painful burns if it touches other tissue, so the first apply a skin barrier around the tissue to be cauterized. Silver nitrate sticks usually need to be moistened with small amount of sterile water to activate. Silver nitrate is applied by running the tip of the stick in a rolling motion over the tissue to be cauterized. Cauterization is usually required 2 to 3 times weekly until granulation tissue resolves.

47. C: Buried bumper syndrome involves migration of the internal bumper into the gastric mucosa. The most common cause is excessive traction pulling the bumper against the gastric mucosa for extended periods, sometimes causing necrotic lesions and abscesses, so there should be 1.5 cm between the external bumper and skin to prevent excessive traction. Symptoms include partial or complete occlusion of the tube, erythema and swelling about stoma, and pain in the abdominal wall. The bumper may be palpable on examination. In all cases, the tube must be removed, either by external traction or surgical excision with endoscopy.

48. D: Prevention of occlusion in enteral feeding tubes requires proper administration of medications and feedings, and maintaining a regular schedule of flushing. Tubes should be flushed with 30 mL of water at least every 4 hours for continuous feeding, as well as before and after intermittent feedings and administration of medications. Medications should be in liquid form or should be crushed completely. Enteric-coated or delayed-release preparations should be avoided, as they may not be adequately absorbed. Feeding solutions should be liquid in consistency.

49. B: The PEG tube does not have an inflatable balloon, but the tube should be stabilized by pulling gently to ensure that the internal bumper is against the abdominal wall and then sliding the external stabilizer to 1.5 cm above the skin. Replacing the PEG tube is done only if the leakage cannot be otherwise controlled. Routine skin care, including application of barrier ointment or other skin sealant, is necessary to prevent skin breakdown. In some cases, alginates, foam dressing, gauze, or pouching may be necessary.

50. D: Because kidneys are active during the night, urinary output may increase to 2 L, so to prevent the ostomy bag from becoming overfull during the night and pulling away from the skin, a long tube should attach a large overnight urinary drainage bag. The bag can be placed in a container on the floor or hung on the side of the bed. Overnight drainage also helps to keep the urine from constantly bathing the stoma, which causes white, gritty crystals to form.

51. B: A patient with an ileostomy has developed hyponatremia when the sodium value drops to less than 135 mEq:

- Normal value: 135-145 mEq/L.
- Hyponatremia: <135 mEq/L. Critical value: <120 mEq/L.
- Hypernatremia: >145 mEq/L. Critical value >160 mEq/L.

Symptoms of hyponatremia may include:

- Irritability to lethargy to confusion and alterations in consciousness.
- Cerebral edema with seizures and coma.
- Dyspnea to respiratory failure.

52. C: A low-profile percutaneous feeding tube is recommended for pediatric patients because it is less likely become dislodged. The low-profile tube is almost flush with the skin whereas the standard tube protrudes up to 7 inches and can easily be pulled out by a child tugging on the tube or catching it on clothing. Adults may also prefer the low-profile tube because it is easier to conceal with clothing and less inconvenient to manage.

53. A: Providing feedback is an essential element of active listening because it shows the speaker that the listener is paying attention and processing what the person is saying as well as paying respect. Feedback may include nodding the head, restating something the person has said, asking pertinent comments, making comments, and showing agreement. The listener should pay close attention to not only the speaker's words but also to nonverbal communication, including gestures, facial expression, body position, and tone of voice.

54. A: Rotating the tube daily is a measure to prevent buried bumper syndrome with a PEG tube. Additionally, the external fixation device should be about 1 to 2 cm above the surface of the skin so that there is no undue tension. If buried bumper syndrome occurs, the patient will likely experience pain, and fluids may infuse poorly. The PEG tube must be removed and replaced if buried bumper syndrome occurs.

55. D: When using a closed suction system to manage a high-output fistula, the suction catheter is positioned next to the fistula orifice but not inside the orifice because of the danger that the catheter may contaminate the fistula and result in ascending infection. The skin about the fistula should be protected with barrier spray and/or hydrocolloid barrier strips and then the wound base is covered with a few layers of moist gauze to protect the tissue from the suction. The catheter is placed on these layers of gauze and covered with additional moist gauze to secure it in place.

56. B: The tract of a PEG usually matures and heals within 2 to 4 weeks. Once the tract has healed, the original PEG tube can generally be replaced with a balloon gastrostomy tube. Gastrostomy tubes with an internal balloon or mushroom tip, measured markings, and an external disk are easier to stabilize, but internal devices should be checked daily by gently pulling until resistance is felt. External stabilizing devices can be applied to the skin to hold the tube in place. The tube may also be taped to the abdomen or secured with a binder.

57. A: If a patient complains of difficulty keeping a seal of an ostomy appliance because of a bulge on one side of the stoma, the most likely cause is parastomal hernia. The hernia may not be always evident unless the patient coughs or strains when it is small, but over time it may enlarge. The patient should be examined in good light in standing, lying, and sitting position and should be asked to cough, lift the head, and strain as though having a bowel movement. Parastomal hernias are usually managed conservatively with diet, flexible pouching system, and hernia support belts.

58. B: Management of severe stomal stenosis usually requires surgical repair. While dilators were used at one time, dilation should not be used long term although digital dilation may be used in an emergent situation. With mild stenosis, dietary modifications may help to relieve symptoms if the stool is kept softer, but dietary modification alone is not generally adequate for severe stenosis.

59. D: If a patient with a colostomy has a new onset of loose stools, the nurse should initially review the patient's food history because, in most cases, loose stools are caused by dietary changes. Foods/Beverages that may increase loose stools include alcohol, beans, cucumbers, fresh fruits, cruciferous vegetables, bran cereals, whole grains, prunes, raisins, raw vegetables, spicy foods, and milk.

60. C: If an ostomy pouch has a drainable spout, it is usually positioned at 6 o'clock so that gravity aids drainage. This position makes it easy to empty the pouch into a toilet while sitting on the toilet or while sitting in front of the toilet. Ostomy pouches with drainable spouts are typically used for urinary ostomy pouches and fecal ostomies with liquid stool, especially with high output.

61. B: An ostomy pouch with a deodorizing gas filter works best with formed stool. A gas filter contains deodorizing charcoal that is sandwiched between breathable membranes. The gas filter is at the top of the appliance where it is less likely to be contaminated with fecal material because moist material may plug the filter and render it useless. The life expectancy of a filter is 24 to 36 hours. For this reason, some patients choose to also add a gas vent to the pouch.

62. A: When preparing a cut-to-fit ostomy pouch, the patient should be taught to trace the stoma on a piece of plastic wrap by placing the plastic wrap directly over the stoma and tracing the outline with a felt-tip pen and then placing the plastic wrap over the cut-to-fit skin barrier and using it as a template to cut the correct size. Sizing templates are available, but they may not be accurate enough if the stoma is irregular-shaped.

63. D: Stomal retraction is most common in patients who are obese although it may also result when the abdominal wall is thick, there is scar tissue, or the mesentery is short. In obese patients, the fatty mesentery interferes with the mobilization of the bowel and puts tension on the stoma, causing it to retract. A retracted stoma increases the risk of leakage under the appliance. A convex pouching system and a belt may help to elevate the stoma.

64. C: A clear pouch should be used over the stoma in the immediate postoperative period in order to allow stomal assessment. The stoma needs to be assessed frequently for early complications, such as mucocutaneous separation, stomal ischemia and necrosis, and stomal retraction as well as signs of bleeding. The patient may or may not be ready to look at the stoma, and the patient should be allowed to proceed at a pace that is right for the individual.

65. B: If the patient is markedly obese with a very large abdomen, the stoma may need to be sited higher than usual because the patient may have difficulty seeing a stoma that is lower on the abdomen. Another consideration is that stomas often retract in obese patients, and the patient may need to wear a belt to secure an appliance. It's important that the appliance avoid creases and the underside of a fold.

66. A: If, following an emergent traumatic injury, a 25-year old patient required a colectomy and permanent end colostomy, but the patient has become increasingly withdrawn and shows evidence of suicidal ideation, the most appropriate response is to refer the patient for psychological counseling. Most patients have some preparation for fecal diversion preoperatively, but the sudden change in body image that may occur with emergent surgery can be difficult for some patients to process and can lead to depression and even suicide. One study indicated that up 60% of patient have considered suicide after colostomy surgery.

67. D: If a patient develops granulomas at the peristomal skin/stoma juncture, the treatment of choice is usually silver nitrate cauterization, which can easily be done in the office or clinic. Cauterization is usually done one to three times a week for about 4 weeks. Small lesions may eventually disappear without treatment, but lesions must be protected from mechanical trauma as they may bleed. Large lesions may require electrical cauterization.

68. D: Sodium phosphate bowel prep is usually more acceptable to patients than polyethylene glycol preparations because sodium phosphate has low volume, so the patient doesn't have to drink so much unpleasant liquid, such as with polyethylene glycol. Polyethylene glycol is an osmotic laxative while sodium phosphate is a hyperosmotic preparation that may result in dehydration and electrolyte imbalance. Sodium phosphate is available in liquid form or in tablets, which must be taken with a prescribed volume of water. Patients should be advised to drink plenty of liquids when taking sodium phosphate and to avoid use of any other laxatives.

69. C: The two primary concerns of ostomy patients are odor control and leakage. Both of these problems can be observed by others, and the patients often feel embarrassed or shame that others may perceive their bodily functions. The nurse should discuss these issues openly with patients and advise them on methods to avoid odor, such as diet control and use of charcoal filters, and leakage and methods to manage them if they do occur.

70. B: When assessing the postoperative condition of a fecal stoma, the nurse expects the stoma to be deep red in color. If the stoma appears pale or dusky, this may be an indication of inadequate oxygenation. Typically, the stoma is initially edematous, but gross edema is cause for concern. The edema subsides over about 6 weeks postoperatively. A stoma that is flush with the skin increases the difficulty of pouching to prevent leakage.

71. B: Ideally, a stoma, such as for an end ileostomy, should protrude from the skin by approximately 2 to 3 centimeters because this allows a pouch to fit snugly about the stoma and decreases the risk that drainage will leak under the appliance and macerate the skin. Also, this allows a little leeway for the normal retraction and extension of the stoma. If the stoma is too long, on the other hand, it is at risk of trauma with increased irritation and bleeding.

72. C: The ideal site for a stoma is in the rectus abdominus muscle. This vertical muscle is in the front of the abdomen, and placing the stoma in this muscle reduces problems, such as parastomal hernias. The incision is made through the muscle longitudinally in the direction of the fibers. The nurse siting the stoma should look for a flat area (at least 8 cm in diameter) within the muscle and in an area free of scars and away from the beltline.

73. D: Following construction of an Indiana pouch, irrigation is usually carried out with 30 to 60 mL normal saline four times daily. Typically, mucus is produced in the pouch and must be flushed out with irrigation. With each irrigation, the procedure should be repeated 3 or more times until the fluid returns clear of mucus. The irrigations are typically spaced throughout the day although this should be guided by the amount of mucus produced and the patency of the catheter.

74. B: The continent ileostomy (Kock pouch) is currently used primarily as a backup for IPAA failure. The Kock pouch is complex to construct and frequently requires revision, so the IPAA has become more commonly used although the Kock pouch may still be utilized for patients who have an inadequate sphincter, have cancer low in the rectum, or do not want an IPAA. Patients with Crohn's disease of the small intestine are not candidates for the Kock pouch.

75. A: The ileal pouch anal anastomosis (IPAA) is not routinely recommended for patients with Crohn's disease because of the increased risk of pouch failure/pouch-associated fistulae. The IPAA can be performed in a one-stage, two-stage, or three-stage procedure. The IPAA procedure removes the colon and the rectum but retains the anal sphincter, and the ileal pouch is formed to serve as the neorectum. In two-stage and three-stage procedures, a temporary ileostomy is created.

76. C: Patients with a perineal wound should be reminded to avoid using a donut cushion because it causes pulling of the incision and decreased blood flow to the area. The patient should be instructed in methods to reduce pressure on the incisional area, such as by shifting weight from one side to the other. Sitz baths or directing the shower at the perineal wound may help to remove drainage and relieve discomfort.

77. D: If a patient with inflammatory bowel disease presents with hair loss, weight loss, balance problems, decreased energy and fatigue, the nurse should suspect malnutrition. Malnutrition is very common in patients with IBD, with the severity correlating to the extent of lesions that interfere with absorption. Patients may have deficiencies in protein and calories as well as micronutrients (vitamins and minerals).

78. B: The most common surgical procedure for Crohn's disease is removal of the terminal ileum and cecum. Surgical resection is usually limited only the area of involvement because lesions often recur and require further surgical intervention, so as much of the intestines as possible is retained. In some cases, primary anastomosis may be done, but if the patient's condition is poor, then a temporary ileostomy may be created to allow healing; however, in many cases, the patient may eventually require an ileostomy.

79. C: With extensive ulcerative colitis, the distance (measured from the anal verge) of involved tissue is greater than 60 cm. Proctitis, which involves generally only the rectum may extend to only 20 cm; left-sided ulcerative colitis extends 35 to 40 cm from the rectum to the splenic flexure; and pancolitis involves the entire colon. The continuous involvement of the tissue is circumferential but involves does not involve the submucosa or muscle layers.

80. A: If a patient with an IPAA experiences anal burning and loose stools after eating certain foods, the treatment may include bile salt binding agents, such as Colestid and cholestyramine, because the burning can likely be attributed to bile salt diarrhea. Foods that tend to trigger burning include those high in fiber/roughage (raw fruits, vegetable, nuts) and acidic foods, such as citrus fruits and tomatoes.

81. D: If a patient has developed skin irritation about a biliary tube, the best solution is to apply alcohol-free liquid skin barrier. Barrier paste contains alcohol and may cause discomfort and further irritation. Barrier pastes with creams and oils should be avoided. The biliary tube must be secured so that it doesn't dislodge and is generally flushed with 10 mL NS twice daily to maintain patency. If blockage occurs, the patient may develop fever, chills, and pain.

82. B: The most common cause of bladder cancer is smoking (cigarettes, cigars, pipes), which accounts for about 50% of cases, and the risk of getting cancer is at least 4 times higher than in non-smokers. While males have a higher overall incidence of bladder cancer, recent studies show the same proportion of females (50%) as males develop bladder cancer related to smoking. Other causes of bladder cancer include exposure to chemicals, history of radiation to the pelvic area, and chronic irritation.

83. C: If siting both a fecal and a urinary stoma, the urinary stoma should be on a different horizontal plane at least one inch higher than the fecal stoma. When siting the stomas, the nurse should consider the surface areas needed for placement of pouches and the patient's possible need to wear an ostomy belt for one or both ostomies to ensure that a belt would not need to cross over the other stoma or pouch.

84. D: A patient with an ileostomy should be advised that the best way to take fluids is immediately after eating because this allows the food to absorb the liquid while it's still in the stomach and slows passage of the liquid into the small bowel. Patients should be encouraged to avoid carbonated beverages (which increase flatus) and beverages with a high sugar content. Recommended drinks include water, Gatorade, coconut water, and vegetable juice (such as V8).

85. B: Chronic pouchitis develops in about 10% of patients with an IPAA. Various factors may be involved in the development of chronic pouchitis, including cytomegalovirus infection, idiopathic, fungal infection, ischemia, bacterial infection (*Escherichia coli*, *Clostridioides difficile*, *Klebsiella*, *Pseudomonas*), NSAID-induced, autoimmune response, spread of Crohn's disease, and cuffitis. Treatment depends on identifying the underlying cause, which may require endoscopy and biopsy.

86. A: If a patient has familial adenomatous polyposis (FAP), the chance of developing colon cancer by age 40 is 100%. FAP is an autosomal dominant disorder resulting from mutation of the APC, a tumor suppressor gene which causes up to thousands of adenomatous polyps to form in the colon and rectum. Cancer may occur at any age, but the average age at diagnosis is 39, most typically in the rectum although the sigmoid and other parts of the colon may be involved. The most common cause of death, however, is periampullary cancer.

87. C: A moderate output enterocutaneous fistula (ECF) is one with output of 200 to 500 mL/24 hours:

- Low output: <200 mL/24 hours.
- Moderate output: 200 to 500 mL/24 hours.
- High output: >500 mL/24 hours.

Output is only one way of categorizing ECFs, as they may also be categorized according to the origin and the etiology. Most ECFs are iatrogenic, with some resulting from leak of an anastomosis and others from trauma associated with surgery.

88. B: Modifiable risk factors for the development of colorectal cancer include high fat/low fat diet. Other modifiable risk factors include lack of exercise and obesity. By making changes in lifestyle, the patient may reduce risk. Non-modifiable risk factors include age (especially older age), disease (such as ulcerative colitis and Crohn's disease), and genetic predisposition.

89. D: If the physician has ordered that a nephrostomy tube be flushed because of mucus and sediment in the urine, the irrigation should be done with 5 to 10 mL of NS. The purpose of flushing is to clear the tube rather than to irrigate the kidney. The saline is instilled into the tube, but not forced, and then drained by gravity. If the tube is so blocked that the saline will not instill, then the physician should be notified immediately.

90. A: Characteristics of ulcerative colitis include superficial mucosal penetration within the colon with continuous areas of involvement but no granulomas or fistulae, perianal disease, or strictures.

Pain is usually minimal, but extraintestinal manifestation may occur. Smoking seems to have some protective function for ulcerative colitis although other negative effects of smoking may occur, so it is not recommended as part of treatment.

91. C: The first step in managing stomal trauma is to identify the cause of the trauma and then to take steps to alleviate the problem. In some cases, the size or type of the pouching system may need to be changed, but trauma may also be caused by other things, such as from the seat belt of a car, from wearing clothing or a belt that is too tight, or from engaging in activities, such as football, that risk direct trauma to the stoma.

92. D: If a patient has a proximal enterocutaneous fistula, the primary concern is nutrition as the proximal location of the origin means that calories, proteins, fluids, and electrolytes are lost in the exudate, which can be copious. Patients may need increased fluids and nutrition to compensate, and in some cases total parental nutrition may be necessary. If the origin is distal, then there may be enough small bowel above the fistula for adequate absorption.

93. C: Most cases of metastatic melanoma to the gastrointestinal system occur in the small intestine with only about 15% in the colon. The primary tumor usually originates from a different site. Patients are often asymptomatic, so the tumor is advanced when it is diagnosed; thus, prognosis is often poor. Treatment includes excision although survival is not prolonged with abdominal perineal resection, so this is usually avoided unless needed to relieve intractable pain.

94. B: A patient with a high output ileostomy should avoid drinking excessive hypotonic fluids, such as water, fruit juice, soda, tea, and coffee because they increase the risk of hyponatremia. These fluids have low sodium content and cause increased loss of sodium in the bowel, and much of this sodium is not reabsorbed, leading to hyponatremia. Patients should be encouraged to drink fluids with electrolytes, such as sports drinks (Gatorade®) or vegetable juices.

95. A: If a patient has an IPAA and has become pregnant, the patient should be advised that she may experience increased frequency of stools and fecal incontinence as the pressure of the fetus bears down on the fecal reservoir. Patients with an IPAA can successfully become pregnant and deliver a healthy infant although whether vaginal delivery or Cesarean is preferred is not yet established, but vaginal delivery may put the anal sphincter more at risk.

96. B: A patient is undergoing video capsule endoscopy for Crohn's disease, a primary concern is capsule retention. For the endoscopy, the patient must swallow a capsule that contains a miniature camera that conveys video imaging to a monitor. In some cases with Crohn's disease, a stricture may develop and the capsule can become imbedded in the strictures and deep endoscopy or surgical intervention is needed in order to remove the capsule.

97. D: If an 80-year-old male is too frail to carry out the irrigations independently and his 72-year-old wife is still confused about the procedure, the best plan is to refer the patient to a home health agency for assistance. The home health nurse can monitor the patient and continue to educate and supervise the patient's wife until she is more comfortable with the irrigation procedures.

98. B: If, when the urostomy appliance is removed after 4 days, the skin is clear but there is erosion in the peristomal area of the barrier of the appliance, this means that the appliance should be changed more frequently because it is starting to break down. This could mean that urine will begin to seep under the barrier and could result in peristomal skin irritation. Most patients change the urostomy bag once or twice a week.

99. A: If a 64-year-old female client has recently had surgery for colon cancer and has a colostomy, but the client has been resistive to educational efforts and refuses to look at the colostomy, the most appropriate intervention is to remain supportive and encourage the client to express her feelings. Clients cope with a changed body image in different ways, and the client may need extra time to process the changes and to cope emotionally.

100. C: If a Vietnamese immigrant patient had surgery for a bowel resection and colostomy but has not requested pain medicine in the 6 hours after returning from the recovery room to his room on the surgical unit, the nurse should assume the patient is reluctant to complain of pain. Asian patients are traditionally stoic, so the nurse should ask the patient to rate or describe his pain rather than asking if the patient has pain.

101. C: When teaching a patient to irrigate a colostomy, the patient should be advised to use 500 to 1000 mL for the irrigation, beginning with 500 mL at first and then adding more fluid until the right amount for the individual is determined. The bag should be filled with 1000 mL warm water and bag hung so that the bottom of the bag is at shoulder level so that gravity will help the flow of water into the bowel. Patients may sit on the toilet with the irrigation bag between the legs or may sit on a chair or stool in front of the toilet.

102. B: The best choice to protect the skin from drainage is skin barrier spray, which provides a thin, breathable layer of silicone protection from both adhesive and discharge (including enzymes). The barrier spray can be applied to the skin prior to application of a wound management/pouching system. The barrier spray does not sting and can be applied quickly because it dries within seconds. (The same product is available in wipes.)

103. D: When siting the stoma for a woman who is 6 months pregnant, the stomas site should be more lateral than the usual site because of the enlarged abdomen. Following pregnancy, when the abdomen returns to a more normal shape, the lateral stoma will move medially. A stoma placed high on the abdomen will tend to shift downward, and a stoma placed low on the abdomen will tend to shift upward.

104. B: Most bacteria that is ingested orally is eliminated by gastric acidity; therefore, the stomach is relatively sterile. However, bacteria increase throughout the small and large intestine. Bile acids in the duodenum and antibodies decrease bacterial growth of aerobic bacteria. Anaerobic bacteria are plentiful distal to the ileocecal valve and serve essential roles in digestion, but they can become pathogenic if the normal balance is disrupted.

105. B: Absorption of nutrients, electrolytes, vitamins, and minerals takes place primarily in the small intestine. Most absorption occurs in the first 100 cm of the small intestine, primarily the duodenum and jejunum, which have plentiful villi. Of the 8 to 9 L of fluid that are received or produced by the small intestine, 7 to 8 L are reabsorbed, including carbohydrates and minerals. The duodenum neutralizes the gastric contents while pancreatic enzymes continue digestion and bile emulsifies fat. Most fats, proteins, and vitamins as well as a smaller amount of carbohydrates are absorbed in the jejunum.

106. C: Penrose drains are usually kept in a wound postoperatively for 3 to 5 days and are usually slowly removed as the wound heals. The drain may be cut with sterile scissors as it is advanced, being sure to place a sterile safety pin near the end to prevent the drain from migrating into the wound. The longer the drain is in place, the greater the risk of developing an ascending infection from the drain.

107. A: Up about 70% of colorectal lymphomas are located in the cecum/ascending colon because this area has a large amount of lymphoid tissue. Onset of symptoms is usually in the 50s to 70s. Because the disease is usually systemic, treatment may include radiation and chemotherapy, but surgery is not usually indicated except for focal lesions or complications, such as perforations. Patients may present with nonspecific symptoms, abdominal pain, and/or abdominal mass

108. D: If a patient is diagnosed with rectal cancer, the TNM (tumor size, nodal status, and metastatic spread) classification that generally indicates the need for transanal excision only is T1N0. T1 indicates that the tumor has invaded the mucosa and the submucosa, and N0 indicates no nodal spread and, therefore, no metastasis. Tis (in situ) would indicate only invasion of the mucosa but not the submucosa.

109. A: Most electrolyte loss occurs through urine because essential electrolytes (sodium, chloride, potassium, calcium, phosphate, bicarbonate, hydrogen, and magnesium) are regulated by the kidneys. Normally, food and food intake provide an adequate electrolyte balance, but disease or surgical interventions (such as ileostomy) may result in electrolyte imbalance that can be life threatening, so the electrolyte balance must be carefully monitored and replacement therapy provided as needed.

110. C: If a colonoscopy shows a fragmented polyp with invasive cancer, the likely treatment will be colectomy, removal of lymph nodes, and possible diversion. If the polyp is not fragmented and is a single specimen that is able to be completely removed, then only observation is needed with colonoscopy at least every 3 years. If colon cancer is found and the lesion is not obstructing, then diversion may or may not be necessary.

111. B: Carcinoid tumors are most common in African Americans. These slow-growing neuroendocrine tumors generally don't occur until the 50s or 60s and are accompanied by carcinoid syndrome in 10% to 18% of patients. Carcinoid syndrome results in flushing of skin, liquid stools, pain in the abdomen, heart failure (right-sided), and wheezing. Colorectal carcinoid tumors are often asymptomatic and found on colonoscopy.

112. D: Smoking makes patients with Crohn's disease more refractory to treatment. Additionally, smokers are more likely to develop Crohn's disease and to exhibit more severe symptoms and may have more than twice as many flareups; therefore, patients with Crohn's disease need to stop smoking as part of the plan of treatment, but they may need support in order to do so. Female patients tend to have more negative effects from smoking than male patients.

113. A: A patient with Crohn's disease is especially at risk for deficiency of vitamin B12 because the terminal ileum, which is essential for vitamin B12 absorption, is the most commonly involved part of the small intestine and the most commonly resected. Patients should receive preventive vitamin B12. If the ileocecal valve and cecum are removed, the patient may also have deficiency of fat-soluble vitamins and zinc.

114. D: With ulcerative colitis, toxic megacolon is an indication for urgent surgery. Other urgent situations include perforation, uncontrolled bleeding, obstruction, and fulminant attack that is nonresponsive to treatment. Indications for elective surgery include refractory disease, adenocarcinoma, failure to thrive (pediatrics), and chronic steroid dependency because delay in surgery is not immediately life threatening.

115. B: If a patient has a subtotal colectomy with ileostomy and a Hartman's pouch for Crohn's disease, the patient should be told to expect to feel the urge to defecate and pass mucus periodically. This usually occurs about once a day because the pouch continues to produce mucus.

With a Hartman's pouch, the anus and rectum stay in place but the top of the rectum is sewn closed. The Hartman's pouch may later be removed if a proctectomy is indicated.

116. A: If a male patient who is 6 weeks postoperative with an IPAA complains of difficulty achieving an erection and engaging in sexual activity and seems quite distressed, the most appropriate referral is to a urologist. During the surgical procedure, sometimes the nerves that affect urination and sexual function become damaged, so the urologist can best make this assessment. In most cases, function resumes within a few months.

117. D: If a patient with Crohn's disease is considering surgery to create an ileostomy, the most important role of the nurse is to provide information about the procedure, including the pros and cons, to help the patient make an informed decision. The nurse could provide literature and pictures to explain the procedure and provide a list of resources, such as the United Ostomy Association of America and Crohn's and Colitis Foundation.

118. B: When a patient undergoing a 3-stage proctocolectomy and IPAA procedure has the end ileostomy changed to a temporary loop ileostomy, the patient is especially at increased risk of dehydration. The loop ileostomy is created more proximally than the end ileostomy, so the stool is very liquid and in large quantities (1000 to 2000 mL/24 hours). Patients should be advised to increase intake of liquids after eating meals and snacks to but avoid drinking on an empty stomach because the fluid will rapidly enter the small intestine.

119. C: If a patient has an ileostomy, the type of food that is most indicated to thicken the stool is starchy foods, which tend to act somewhat like a sponge and absorb liquid. Starchy foods include potatoes, rice, and foods made with flour, such as bread and pasta. Sugary foods are also high in starch, but the calories provide little in the way of nutrition, and since malnutrition is always a concern, they should be avoided.

120. A: A contradiction to negative pressure wound therapy (NPWT) (AKA vacuum-assisted wound closure) for an enterocutaneous fistula is an exposed bowel at the wound base because the suction may result in perforation of the bowel. The tract must have the potential for spontaneous closure, so NPWT is contraindicated if a pseudostoma is evident. NPWT should not be used for a fistula if an abscess is present or if there is a distal obstruction and should be avoided if malignancy is present.

How to Overcome Test Anxiety

Just the thought of taking a test is enough to make most people a little nervous. A test is an important event that can have a long-term impact on your future, so it's important to take it seriously and it's natural to feel anxious about performing well. But just because anxiety is normal, that doesn't mean that it's helpful in test taking, or that you should simply accept it as part of your life. Anxiety can have a variety of effects. These effects can be mild, like making you feel slightly nervous, or severe, like blocking your ability to focus or remember even a simple detail.

If you experience test anxiety—whether severe or mild—it's important to know how to beat it. To discover this, first you need to understand what causes test anxiety.

Causes of Test Anxiety

While we often think of anxiety as an uncontrollable emotional state, it can actually be caused by simple, practical things. One of the most common causes of test anxiety is that a person does not feel adequately prepared for their test. This feeling can be the result of many different issues such as poor study habits or lack of organization, but the most common culprit is time management. Starting to study too late, failing to organize your study time to cover all of the material, or being distracted while you study will mean that you're not well prepared for the test. This may lead to cramming the night before, which will cause you to be physically and mentally exhausted for the test. Poor time management also contributes to feelings of stress, fear, and hopelessness as you realize you are not well prepared but don't know what to do about it.

Other times, test anxiety is not related to your preparation for the test but comes from unresolved fear. This may be a past failure on a test, or poor performance on tests in general. It may come from comparing yourself to others who seem to be performing better or from the stress of living up to expectations. Anxiety may be driven by fears of the future—how failure on this test would affect your educational and career goals. These fears are often completely irrational, but they can still negatively impact your test performance.

Elements of Test Anxiety

As mentioned earlier, test anxiety is considered to be an emotional state, but it has physical and mental components as well. Sometimes you may not even realize that you are suffering from test anxiety until you notice the physical symptoms. These can include trembling hands, rapid heartbeat, sweating, nausea, and tense muscles. Extreme anxiety may lead to fainting or vomiting. Obviously, any of these symptoms can have a negative impact on testing. It is important to recognize them as soon as they begin to occur so that you can address the problem before it damages your performance.

The mental components of test anxiety include trouble focusing and inability to remember learned information. During a test, your mind is on high alert, which can help you recall information and stay focused for an extended period of time. However, anxiety interferes with your mind's natural processes, causing you to blank out, even on the questions you know well. The strain of testing during anxiety makes it difficult to stay focused, especially on a test that may take several hours. Extreme anxiety can take a huge mental toll, making it difficult not only to recall test information but even to understand the test questions or pull your thoughts together.

Effects of Test Anxiety

Test anxiety is like a disease—if left untreated, it will get progressively worse. Anxiety leads to poor performance, and this reinforces the feelings of fear and failure, which in turn lead to poor performances on subsequent tests. It can grow from a mild nervousness to a crippling condition. If allowed to progress, test anxiety can have a big impact on your schooling, and consequently on your future.

Test anxiety can spread to other parts of your life. Anxiety on tests can become anxiety in any stressful situation, and blanking on a test can turn into panicking in a job situation. But fortunately, you don't have to let anxiety rule your testing and determine your grades. There are a number of relatively simple steps you can take to move past anxiety and function normally on a test and in the rest of life.

Physical Steps for Beating Test Anxiety

While test anxiety is a serious problem, the good news is that it can be overcome. It doesn't have to control your ability to think and remember information. While it may take time, you can begin taking steps today to beat anxiety.

Just as your first hint that you may be struggling with anxiety comes from the physical symptoms, the first step to treating it is also physical. Rest is crucial for having a clear, strong mind. If you are tired, it is much easier to give in to anxiety. But if you establish good sleep habits, your body and mind will be ready to perform optimally, without the strain of exhaustion. Additionally, sleeping well helps you to retain information better, so you're more likely to recall the answers when you see the test questions.

Getting good sleep means more than going to bed on time. It's important to allow your brain time to relax. Take study breaks from time to time so it doesn't get overworked, and don't study right before bed. Take time to rest your mind before trying to rest your body, or you may find it difficult to fall asleep.

Along with sleep, other aspects of physical health are important in preparing for a test. Good nutrition is vital for good brain function. Sugary foods and drinks may give a burst of energy but this burst is followed by a crash, both physically and emotionally. Instead, fuel your body with protein and vitamin-rich foods.

Also, drink plenty of water. Dehydration can lead to headaches and exhaustion, especially if your brain is already under stress from the rigors of the test. Particularly if your test is a long one, drink water during the breaks. And if possible, take an energy-boosting snack to eat between sections.

Along with sleep and diet, a third important part of physical health is exercise. Maintaining a steady workout schedule is helpful, but even taking 5-minute study breaks to walk can help get your blood pumping faster and clear your head. Exercise also releases endorphins, which contribute to a positive feeling and can help combat test anxiety.

When you nurture your physical health, you are also contributing to your mental health. If your body is healthy, your mind is much more likely to be healthy as well. So take time to rest, nourish your body with healthy food and water, and get moving as much as possible. Taking these physical steps will make you stronger and more able to take the mental steps necessary to overcome test anxiety.

Mental Steps for Beating Test Anxiety

Working on the mental side of test anxiety can be more challenging, but as with the physical side, there are clear steps you can take to overcome it. As mentioned earlier, test anxiety often stems from lack of preparation, so the obvious solution is to prepare for the test. Effective studying may be the most important weapon you have for beating test anxiety, but you can and should employ several other mental tools to combat fear.

First, boost your confidence by reminding yourself of past success—tests or projects that you aced. If you're putting as much effort into preparing for this test as you did for those, there's no reason you should expect to fail here. Work hard to prepare; then trust your preparation.

Second, surround yourself with encouraging people. It can be helpful to find a study group, but be sure that the people you're around will encourage a positive attitude. If you spend time with others who are anxious or cynical, this will only contribute to your own anxiety. Look for others who are motivated to study hard from a desire to succeed, not from a fear of failure.

Third, reward yourself. A test is physically and mentally tiring, even without anxiety, and it can be helpful to have something to look forward to. Plan an activity following the test, regardless of the outcome, such as going to a movie or getting ice cream.

When you are taking the test, if you find yourself beginning to feel anxious, remind yourself that you know the material. Visualize successfully completing the test. Then take a few deep, relaxing breaths and return to it. Work through the questions carefully but with confidence, knowing that you are capable of succeeding.

Developing a healthy mental approach to test taking will also aid in other areas of life. Test anxiety affects more than just the actual test—it can be damaging to your mental health and even contribute to depression. It's important to beat test anxiety before it becomes a problem for more than testing.

Study Strategy

Being prepared for the test is necessary to combat anxiety, but what does being prepared look like? You may study for hours on end and still not feel prepared. What you need is a strategy for test prep. The next few pages outline our recommended steps to help you plan out and conquer the challenge of preparation.

Step 1: Scope Out the Test

Learn everything you can about the format (multiple choice, essay, etc.) and what will be on the test. Gather any study materials, course outlines, or sample exams that may be available. Not only will this help you to prepare, but knowing what to expect can help to alleviate test anxiety.

Step 2: Map Out the Material

Look through the textbook or study guide and make note of how many chapters or sections it has. Then divide these over the time you have. For example, if a book has 15 chapters and you have five days to study, you need to cover three chapters each day. Even better, if you have the time, leave an extra day at the end for overall review after you have gone through the material in depth.

If time is limited, you may need to prioritize the material. Look through it and make note of which sections you think you already have a good grasp on, and which need review. While you are studying, skim quickly through the familiar sections and take more time on the challenging parts.

Write out your plan so you don't get lost as you go. Having a written plan also helps you feel more in control of the study, so anxiety is less likely to arise from feeling overwhelmed at the amount to cover.

Step 3: Gather Your Tools

Decide what study method works best for you. Do you prefer to highlight in the book as you study and then go back over the highlighted portions? Or do you type out notes of the important information? Or is it helpful to make flashcards that you can carry with you? Assemble the pens, index cards, highlighters, post-it notes, and any other materials you may need so you won't be distracted by getting up to find things while you study.

If you're having a hard time retaining the information or organizing your notes, experiment with different methods. For example, try color-coding by subject with colored pens, highlighters, or post-it notes. If you learn better by hearing, try recording yourself reading your notes so you can listen while in the car, working out, or simply sitting at your desk. Ask a friend to quiz you from your flashcards, or try teaching someone the material to solidify it in your mind.

Step 4: Create Your Environment

It's important to avoid distractions while you study. This includes both the obvious distractions like visitors and the subtle distractions like an uncomfortable chair (or a too-comfortable couch that makes you want to fall asleep). Set up the best study environment possible: good lighting and a comfortable work area. If background music helps you focus, you may want to turn it on, but otherwise keep the room quiet. If you are using a computer to take notes, be sure you don't have any other windows open, especially applications like social media, games, or anything else that could distract you. Silence your phone and turn off notifications. Be sure to keep water close by so you stay hydrated while you study (but avoid unhealthy drinks and snacks).

Also, take into account the best time of day to study. Are you freshest first thing in the morning? Try to set aside some time then to work through the material. Is your mind clearer in the afternoon or evening? Schedule your study session then. Another method is to study at the same time of day that you will take the test, so that your brain gets used to working on the material at that time and will be ready to focus at test time.

Step 5: Study!

Once you have done all the study preparation, it's time to settle into the actual studying. Sit down, take a few moments to settle your mind so you can focus, and begin to follow your study plan. Don't give in to distractions or let yourself procrastinate. This is your time to prepare so you'll be ready to fearlessly approach the test. Make the most of the time and stay focused.

Of course, you don't want to burn out. If you study too long you may find that you're not retaining the information very well. Take regular study breaks. For example, taking five minutes out of every hour to walk briskly, breathing deeply and swinging your arms, can help your mind stay fresh.

As you get to the end of each chapter or section, it's a good idea to do a quick review. Remind yourself of what you learned and work on any difficult parts. When you feel that you've mastered the material, move on to the next part. At the end of your study session, briefly skim through your notes again.

But while review is helpful, cramming last minute is NOT. If at all possible, work ahead so that you won't need to fit all your study into the last day. Cramming overloads your brain with more information than it can process and retain, and your tired mind may struggle to recall even previously learned information when it is overwhelmed with last-minute study. Also, the urgent nature of cramming and the stress placed on your brain contribute to anxiety. You'll be more likely to go to the test feeling unprepared and having trouble thinking clearly.

So don't cram, and don't stay up late before the test, even just to review your notes at a leisurely pace. Your brain needs rest more than it needs to go over the information again. In fact, plan to finish your studies by noon or early afternoon the day before the test. Give your brain the rest of the day to relax or focus on other things, and get a good night's sleep. Then you will be fresh for the test and better able to recall what you've studied.

Step 6: Take a Practice Test

Many courses offer sample tests, either online or in the study materials. This is an excellent resource to check whether you have mastered the material, as well as to prepare for the test format and environment.

Check the test format ahead of time: the number of questions, the type (multiple choice, free response, etc.), and the time limit. Then create a plan for working through them. For example, if you have 30 minutes to take a 60-question test, your limit is 30 seconds per question. Spend less time on the questions you know well so that you can take more time on the difficult ones.

If you have time to take several practice tests, take the first one open book, with no time limit. Work through the questions at your own pace and make sure you fully understand them. Gradually work up to taking a test under test conditions: sit at a desk with all study materials put away and set a timer. Pace yourself to make sure you finish the test with time to spare and go back to check your answers if you have time.

After each test, check your answers. On the questions you missed, be sure you understand why you missed them. Did you misread the question (tests can use tricky wording)? Did you forget the information? Or was it something you hadn't learned? Go back and study any shaky areas that the practice tests reveal.

Taking these tests not only helps with your grade, but also aids in combating test anxiety. If you're already used to the test conditions, you're less likely to worry about it, and working through tests until you're scoring well gives you a confidence boost. Go through the practice tests until you feel comfortable, and then you can go into the test knowing that you're ready for it.

Test Tips

On test day, you should be confident, knowing that you've prepared well and are ready to answer the questions. But aside from preparation, there are several test day strategies you can employ to maximize your performance.

First, as stated before, get a good night's sleep the night before the test (and for several nights before that, if possible). Go into the test with a fresh, alert mind rather than staying up late to study.

Try not to change too much about your normal routine on the day of the test. It's important to eat a nutritious breakfast, but if you normally don't eat breakfast at all, consider eating just a protein bar. If you're a coffee drinker, go ahead and have your normal coffee. Just make sure you time it so that the caffeine doesn't wear off right in the middle of your test. Avoid sugary beverages, and drink enough water to stay hydrated but not so much that you need a restroom break 10 minutes into the test. If your test isn't first thing in the morning, consider going for a walk or doing a light workout before the test to get your blood flowing.

Allow yourself enough time to get ready, and leave for the test with plenty of time to spare so you won't have the anxiety of scrambling to arrive in time. Another reason to be early is to select a good seat. It's helpful to sit away from doors and windows, which can be distracting. Find a good seat, get out your supplies, and settle your mind before the test begins.

When the test begins, start by going over the instructions carefully, even if you already know what to expect. Make sure you avoid any careless mistakes by following the directions.

Then begin working through the questions, pacing yourself as you've practiced. If you're not sure on an answer, don't spend too much time on it, and don't let it shake your confidence. Either skip it and come back later, or eliminate as many wrong answers as possible and guess among the remaining ones. Don't dwell on these questions as you continue—put them out of your mind and focus on what lies ahead.

Be sure to read all of the answer choices, even if you're sure the first one is the right answer. Sometimes you'll find a better one if you keep reading. But don't second-guess yourself if you do immediately know the answer. Your gut instinct is usually right. Don't let test anxiety rob you of the information you know.

If you have time at the end of the test (and if the test format allows), go back and review your answers. Be cautious about changing any, since your first instinct tends to be correct, but make sure you didn't misread any of the questions or accidentally mark the wrong answer choice. Look over any you skipped and make an educated guess.

At the end, leave the test feeling confident. You've done your best, so don't waste time worrying about your performance or wishing you could change anything. Instead, celebrate the successful completion of this test. And finally, use this test to learn how to deal with anxiety even better next time.

Review Video: Test Anxiety
Visit mometrix.com/academy and enter code: 100340

Important Qualification

Not all anxiety is created equal. If your test anxiety is causing major issues in your life beyond the classroom or testing center, or if you are experiencing troubling physical symptoms related to your anxiety, it may be a sign of a serious physiological or psychological condition. If this sounds like your situation, we strongly encourage you to seek professional help.

Online Resources

Due to our efforts to try to keep this book to a manageable length, we've created a link that will give you access to all of your online resources:

mometrix.com/resources719/cocn

It's Your Moment, Let's Celebrate It!

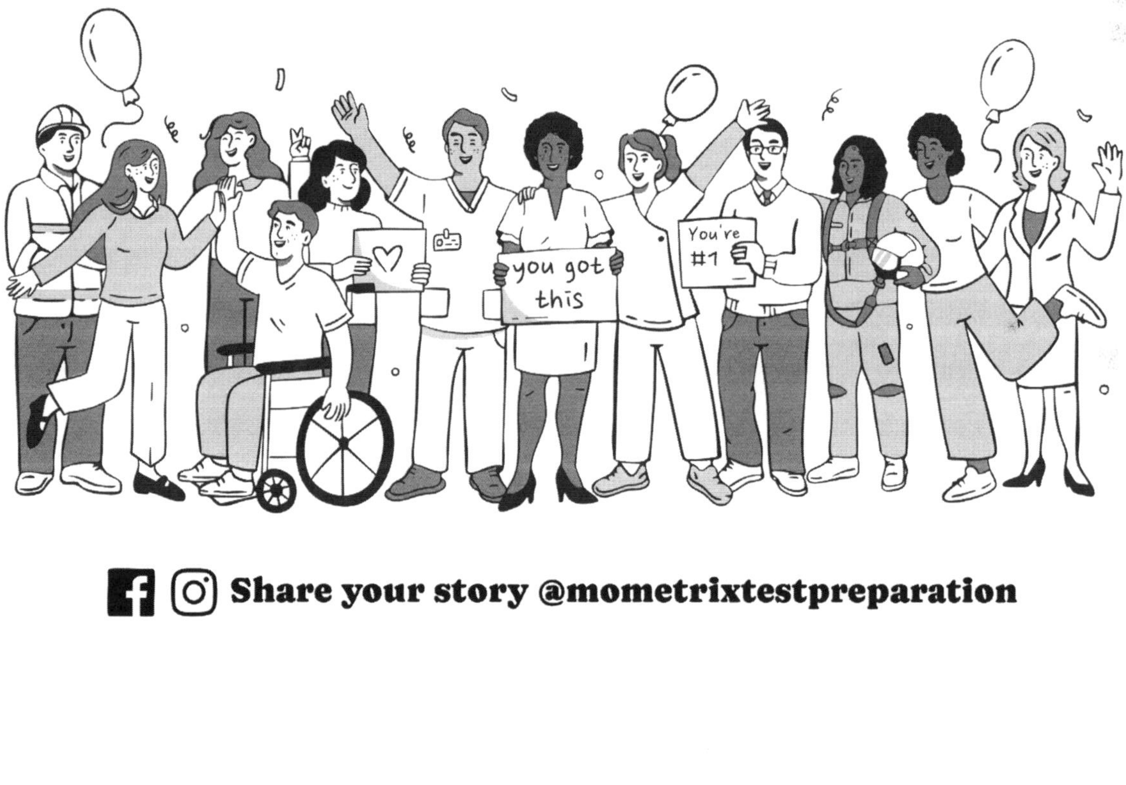

Share your story @mometrixtestpreparation